AF449453

# Issues in Infectious Diseases

## Vol. 6

Series Editor

**Brian W.J. Mahy** Atlanta, Ga.

# Antimicrobial Resistance

## Beyond the Breakpoint

Volume Editor

J. Todd Weber Stockholm

4 figures and 18 tables, 2010

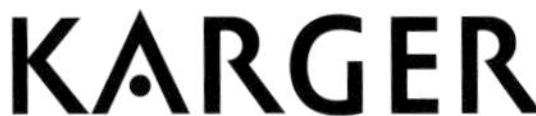

Basel · Freiburg · Paris · London · New York · Bangalore · Bangkok · Shanghai · Singapore · Tokyo · Sydney

**Issues in Infectious Diseases**

**J. Todd Weber**
U.S. Centers for Disease Control
and Prevention
c/o European Centre for Disease
Prevention and Control
171 83 Stockholm (Sweden)

Library of Congress Cataloging-in-Publication Data

Antimicrobial resistance : beyond the breakpoint / volume editor, J. Todd
Weber.
   p. ; cm. -- (Issues in infectious diseases, ISSN 1660-1890 ; v. 6)
  Includes bibliographical references and index.
  ISBN 978-3-8055-9323-6 (hard cover : alk. paper)
  1. Drug resistance in microorganisms. I. Weber, J. Todd. II. Series:
Issues in infectious diseases, v. 6. 1660-1890 ;
  [DNLM: 1. Drug Resistance, Microbial. QW 45 A6306 2010]
  QR177.A5855 2010
  616.9'041--dc22
              2009049841

# Contents

# Foreword

This volume in the series *Issues in Infectious Diseases* deals with one of the most important topics in the field: antimicrobial resistance.

Since antimicrobial drugs were first discovered and used during the Second World War, they have saved countless lives and eased the suffering of millions of people. Unfortunately, in recent years we have seen the emergence and spread of microbes that have acquired resistance to many of the antibiotics in widespread use. Some of the most important of these are penicillin-resistant *Streptococcus pneumoniae*, vancomycin-resistant enterococci, multidrug-resistant salmonellae and *Mycobacterium tuberculosis*, and methicillin-resistant *Staphylococcus aureus* (commonly known as MRSA).

The consequences of infection with these widespread antibiotic-resistant microbes have led to patients fearing to enter hospitals, since medical facilities are often sources of such microbes.

In this, the sixth volume of this series, we consider the full scale of the costs of antimicrobial resistance to our society, both in human and economic terms.

*Brian W.J. Mahy*
Centers for Disease Control and Prevention, Atlanta, Ga.

# Preface

> One characteristic which streptomycin seems unfortunately to share with many antibiotics is that of rapidly inducing in susceptible organisms a high resistance to the drug. This is a subject which obviously offers interesting prospects for analysis.
>
> Sir Howard W. Florey
> Penicillin
> Nobel Lecture, December 11, 1945

Florey was instrumental in launching the antibiotic era and his observations are as true now as they were then. In 2009, the Royal Swedish Academy of Sciences awarded the Nobel Prize in Chemistry to Venkatraman Ramakrishnan, Thomas A. Steitz and Ada E. Yonath 'for studies of the structure and function of the ribosome'. Their work included the creation of three-dimensional models used by scientists to develop new antibiotics, which the Royal Academy said had directly assisted in saving lives and decreasing humanity's suffering. However, we can anticipate that microbes will develop resistance to any new antimicrobial drugs developed on the basis of this or another scientific discovery, eventually making the drugs powerless against one, many or all infections.

At the most simple and definitional level, resistance is the numerical value generated by susceptibility testing to determine whether a microorganism meets criteria for being 'susceptible', 'intermediate' or 'resistant' to an antimicrobial drug. These terms are colloquially referred to as 'breakpoints'. But the real measure of impact is the ability to cure infections and improve the health of patients. Antimicrobial (or, synonymously, antibiotic) resistance has cut a swath through the effectiveness of all antimicrobial classes used to treat infectious diseases. Listing the combinations of drugs and their counterpart resistant pathogens would be a volume in itself. However, for bacteria important examples include the aminoglycosides (resistance in *Acinetobacter baumannii* and *Pseudomonas aeruginosa* causing infections in critically ill patients), aminopenicillins (resistance in community-acquired infections and *Enterococcus* spp. that cause bloodstream infections in hospitalized patients), carbapenems (resistance in *Klebsiella pneumoniae* that causes healthcare-associated infections), quinolones (resistance in various Gram-negative and Gram-positive bacteria such as *Escherichia coli* causing urinary tract infections and *Neisseria gonorrhoeae* causing sexual transmitted infections), cephalosporins (resistance in various Gram-negative and Gram-positive bacteria associated with community- and healthcare-associated infections), antipseudomonal cephalosporins (resistance in *Pseudomonas aeruginosa*), macrolides (resistance in pneumonia and meningitis caused by *Streptococcus pneumoniae*), and anti-staphylococcal semi-synthetic penicillins (resistance in *Staphylococcus aureus* causing community-associated and healthcare-associated skin and soft-tissue infections including surgical-site infections).

In addition, there is ubiquitous antimalarial resistance that has hampered malaria treatment and prophylaxis worldwide, anti-tuberculous drug resistance that has forced longer and more toxic regimens against tuberculosis, antiretroviral resistance in HIV requiring increasingly complex regimens, and antiviral resistance among seasonal influenza strains further reducing already limited treatment options. If we are willing to include the visible among the category of 'microbes', increasing resistance of lice (*Pediculus humanus capitis*) to treatment should also be noted.

This volume does not address the very important problem of the paucity of new antimicrobial drugs and drug classes in the pharmaceutical pipeline. If this pipeline had been full and flowing in recent years, there would be less concern over resistance to older drugs. Instead, there have been few new antimicrobial drugs developed, even fewer new classes, and several large pharmaceutical companies have abandoned research and development in the area of antibacterial drugs.

The authors of these chapters have focused on issues in various aspects of antimicrobial resistance that challenge our ability to slow its inexorable progress, and how we can make the best use of the effectiveness of currently available antimicrobials. Miller examines the changing epidemiology of methicillin-resistant *S. aureus* that is creating diagnostic challenges and forcing the creation of new prevention strategies. Paterson and Doi describe the detection dilemmas and dwindling choices of antimicrobial drugs for critically ill patients infected with these organisms. Parry details the explosive increase in the use of fluoroquinolones for a wide range of diseases and the equally wide ranging resistance consequences, including food-borne pathogens and sexually transmitted infections. Moore and Whitney provide timely analysis of the role of secondary bacterial pneumonia in the context of an influenza pandemic and likelihood that resistant pathogens will play a role in the current pandemic. Belongia et al. summarize the evidence for the methods that effectively reduce the unnecessary use of antimicrobial drugs in the community, a principal tool for slowing the spread of antimicrobial resistance. Similarly, Rezai and Weinstein present the evidence for methods to prevent the spread of antimicrobial-resistant infections in healthcare settings. In a closely related chapter, Merz et al. review the data for the cost of antimicrobial resistance in healthcare settings, providing some of the information needed to convince healthcare institutions to invest more in infection control. Churcher et al. look at the necessary strategy of mass treatment to control parasitic disease and what impact this can have on anthelmintic resistance. Arthington-Skaggs and Frade present the difficulty in measuring resistance in fungal pathogens and the ambiguous relationship of in vitro findings with patient response to treatment. Bennett dissects the threat of resistance that has been used to argue against bringing effective anti-retroviral regimens to much of the world's HIV-infected population.

As Bennett notes for the example of HIV, the fear of resistance should not deter the appropriate use of antimicrobial drugs to reduce morbidity and to save lives. Resistance is an inevitable consequence of even the most perfect use of antimicrobial drugs. Appropriate use combined with prevention strategies described in this volume are the tools we must adhere to now and in the future for the health of our patients.

*J. Todd Weber*, Stockholm

Weber JT (ed): Antimicrobial Resistance – Beyond the Breakpoint.
Issues Infect Dis. Basel, Karger, 2010, vol 6, pp 1–20

# Community-Associated Methicillin Resistant *Staphylococcus aureus*

Loren Gregory Miller

David Geffen School of Medicine at UCLA, Division of Infectious Diseases, Harbor-UCLA Medical Center, Torrance, Calif., USA

### Abstract

Community-associated methicillin-resistant *Staphylococcus aureus* has rapidly risen in incidence to become not only very common, but the predominant cause of *S. aureus* infections in many parts of the world. This bacterium is notable for its predilection to cause infections in healthy persons and be transmitted easily from person to person. Additionally, this organism has the ability to cause severe, life-threatening infections that were previously only rarely, if ever, associated with *S. aureus*. Optimal methods to treat and prevent this infection are uncertain and will require extensive investigation.

Copyright © 2010 S. Karger AG, Basel

Infections caused by community-associated methicillin-resistant *Staphylococcus aureus* (CA-MRSA) have, in a relatively brief period of time, been transformed from a rare entity worthy of case reports, to a common infection. In many parts of the world CA-MRSA infections are common reasons that patients present to primary care physicians, urgent care clinics, and emergency departments. CA-MRSA infections are also being seen increasingly by subspecialty practitioners, who previously had not encountered or were not aware that community-associated *S. aureus* infections could be and are caused by MRSA. This chapter will review current understanding of the epidemiology, pathogenesis, treatment and prevention of CA-MRSA infections.

### *S. aureus*, MRSA and Community-Associated Infections: Background

*S. aureus* is a ubiquitous human pathogen and a common cause of invasive and life-threatening infections. It is the most common cause of community-associated cellulitis [1, 2] and endocarditis [3], and is a common cause of bacteremia [1, 4, 5]. *S. aureus* strains were once nearly uniformly susceptible to semi-synthetic penicillinase-resistant β-lactams (e.g. methicillin, oxacillin), the most commonly used class of antibiotics for skin infection. These strains were termed 'methicillin resistant *Staphylococcus aureus,*' or MRSA, a term that implied cross-resistance to all β-lactams including all penicillins and cephalosporins. By the 1970s, MRSA outbreaks were reported in large, urban, tertiary care hospitals in the United States. Soon MRSA became endemic as a nosocomial pathogen in many hospitals [6]. MRSA infections acquired in the community, however, remained extremely rare.

Defining a 'community-associated' infection is challenging. Most experts prefer the term 'community-associated' rather than other terms found in the literature (e.g. community-acquired, community-onset). In the past, terms such as 'nosocomially acquired' and 'community-acquired' were used to describe the locale in which an infection was acquired. More recently, public health officials have emphasized describing the origin of the organism that subsequently caused the infection (community vs. healthcare setting) rather than just where the infection was acquired [7].

Many CA-MRSA definitions have been used [8]. One commonly used definition of community-associated is based on epidemiologic risk factors. The designation of MRSA as CA-MRSA infection reflects that the MRSA culture was obtained in the outpatient setting or isolated during 72 h of hospitalization *and* the patient did not have exposures associated with healthcare-associated (HA) MRSA infections, such as recent (defined as 'in the prior 12 months') hospitalization, receipt of hemodialysis, residence in a chronic care facility, or presence of an indwelling catheter [9].

Others have used molecular characteristics of the MRSA isolate to distinguish CA-MRSA from HA-MRSA strains. CA-MRSA infections are typically caused by strains that carry Staphylococcal Chromosomal Cassette (SCC)*mec* type IV (or V), whereas HA-MRSA is typically caused by strains that contain SCC*mec* types I–III (discussed below). However, a molecular definition of CA-MRSA is limiting. The rule that MRSA containing SCC*mec* type IV causes community-associated infections is increasingly being violated. Many groups have reported SCC*mec* type IV-containing MRSA strains causing healthcare-associated infections [10–12]. In one hospital in Los Angeles, SCC*mec* type IV-containing MRSA is now responsible for the majority of HA-MRSA infections, surpassing SCC*mec* types I–III in prevalence [12]. An epidemiologic definition of CA-MRSA is more advantageous as strains of both community- and healthcare-associated *S. aureus* are known to evolve over time [13].

Nevertheless, any epidemiologic classification system has limitations. For example, patients with exposures that would categorize their infection as healthcare-associated (e.g. hospitalization in the prior year), but have an MRSA infection almost certainly associated with an outbreak (e.g. in a prison or among football players) would incorrectly have their infection categorized as a HA-MRSA infection. Others have noted that rates of CA-MRSA versus HA-MRSA can vary dramatically depending on the definitions and data source used to determine community-associated status. These miscategorizations may distract investigators from potentially important healthcare sources of infection [14].

**Rapid Increase in CA-MRSA Incidence**

The incidence of CA-MRSA infections and reported numbers of outbreaks has increased at a rapid rate during the late 1990s and the early 21st century. Retrospective investigations of Native Americans in rural areas of the Midwestern United States [15] and of hospitalized children in Chicago [16] demonstrated 15-fold and 7-fold increases, respectively, in the proportion of community-associated *S. aureus* isolates that were methicillin-resistant during the 1990s. In the latter study, the proportion of children with *S. aureus* infections caused by CA-MRSA more than doubled, from 25–67%, over a 5-year period. This rise was due to a 26-fold increase in the incidence of MRSA in infected children with no recognized risk factors for MRSA. Similarly, a retrospective study from Texas found a 7-fold increase in the incidence of CA-MRSA infections from 1997–2000 relative to 1990–1996 [17].

In a similar time period, outbreaks of CA-MRSA infection have been increasingly described. Many populations of healthy persons have been affected. These populations include inmates in jails and prisons [18, 19], athletes participating in contact sports [18, 20], military personnel [21, 22], HIV-infected men who have sex with men [23, 24], and intravenous drug users [8, 25], among other populations. Outbreaks of CA-MRSA are being reported worldwide, including in the United States, Europe, Australia and Asia [26]. In many parts of the world, CA-MRSA infections are endemic and not associated with recognized outbreaks. Several centers have shown that MRSA is responsible for over 50% of community-associated *S. aureus* infections [27, 28].

**Risk Factors, Clinical Manifestations and Transmission**

Risk factors for CA-MRSA infection among the general population are incompletely understood. Data on CA-MRSA risk factors often come from outbreak investigations, which typically occur in relatively homogenous patient populations, such as inmates and athletes [28]. Studies on risk factors for endemic CA-MRSA infections (i.e. infections occurring in non-outbreak settings) frequently come from single centers, making findings difficult to extrapolate to other locales. That said, there are a few commonalities in studies of risk factors. Ethnic minorities comprise 50–90% of CA-MRSA patients in several case series [29–31], and lower socioeconomic status has been associated with increased CA-MRSA risk as well [30, 31]. In several investigations, drug use (typically via an intravenous route) is a significant risk factor for MRSA infection [28, 32–34]. A large study investigation conducted in 3 metropolitan centers in the United Sates found that those of African-American race and those under 2 years of age had higher incidences of CA-MRSA infection [35]. A single-center case-control investigation comparing detailed behaviors of those with and without CA-MRSA infections found that persons with CA-MRSA infection were more likely to report skin breaks, high risk sexual behavior, recent contact with someone with a skin infection, snorting or injecting illegal drugs, recent incarceration, homelessness, and visiting bars, raves or clubs [33].

The vast majority (>80–90%) of CA-MRSA infections manifest as skin and soft tissue infections [24, 28, 29, 36]. Skin infection manifestations include abscess, furuncles and boils. Many patients suffer from recurrent CA-MRSA skin infections [37–40]. Disturbingly, CA-MRSA has caused less common but very serious invasive infections. These infections include necrotizing pneumonia, necrotizing fasciitis, a septic shock syndrome characterized by multi-organ involvement among children, Waterhouse-Friderichsen syndrome, purpura fulminans, myositis, deep-seated infections of bone and joints, septic thrombophlebitis with extensive pulmonary embolization, and other serious syndromes [41]. Although some of these invasive disease syndromes had been described with methicillin-susceptible *S. aureus* (MSSA), many had not previously been reported to be associated with *S. aureus* and they appear been more frequently associated with CA-MRSA. Most of the syndromes are associated with genes for toxins, such as *pvl* (see below), that are commonly found in CA-MRSA strains but are rare among HA-MRSA strains.

Transmission of CA-MRSA strains and infections to close contacts, including those in the same household, has been commonly reported. A Taiwanese study found that 21% of household members, school classmates and schoolteachers of an adolescent who suffered from a serious CA-MRSA infection were colonized with CA-MRSA, many with the same strain as the index patient [42]. Among children attending 2 daycare centers in Dallas, 3 and 12%, respectively, were colonized with MRSA of the same type (as determined by pulsed-field gel electrophoresis) as index cases hospitalized with CA-MRSA infection [31]. Another study showed that 16% of patients with CA-MRSA skin infections had a close contact with another person with a skin infection in the past month compared to 7% of CA-MSSA patients [28]. Finally, a prospective study showed that among patients with community-associated *S. aureus* infections, 30 days after diagnosis, reports of new skin infection among household members was 13% for CA-MRSA patients but just 4% for those who had CA-MSSA, although this did not achieve statistical significance (p = 0.20) [43]. Because CA-MRSA infections have only recently emerged, the rate of transmission of CA-MRSA infections to household members are still not well quantified. Nevertheless, it is common for investigators and clinicians to comment on the high rate of CA-MRSA infection among close contacts [37].

When comparing patients with CA-MRSA and CA-MSSA infections, 'risk factors' such as recent hospitalization, receipt of hemodialysis, recent incarceration, illicit drug use or participation in contact sports are too unreliable to distinguish MRSA infection [28]. Therefore, among patients with community-associated *S. aureus* infection, simply lacking the above MRSA risk factors is insufficient to exclude MRSA since many patients with the infection have none of these risks [27, 28]. Because CA-MRSA appears to be able infect virtually anyone, in locales where CA-MRSA is seen community-associated *S. aureus* infections should be suspected to be MRSA until proven otherwise (e.g. by standard tests performed at clinical microbiology laboratories).

## Differences between CA-MRSA and HA-MRSA

When contrasting CA-MRSA and HA-MRSA infections and strains, several differences have been noted. First, HA-MRSA isolates are typically resistant to multiple non-β-lactam antimicrobials. However, CA-MRSA isolates are usually susceptible to many non-β-lactam antibiotics, including trimethoprim-sulfamethoxazole, clindamycin and tetracyclines [44–46]. Second, several severe clinical syndromes have been associated with CA-MRSA isolates that are less well described in association with HA-MRSA isolates. Third, the expression of toxins in CA-MRSA isolates such as Panton-Valentine leukocidin (PVL), a pore-forming toxin causing lysis of several mammalian cell lines, may be responsible for certain novel clinical features of CA-MRSA disease at the severe end of the clinical spectrum, although the role of PVL remains controversial at this time.

A survey of toxin genes known to be present in sequenced *S. aureus* strains has demonstrated important differences between CA-MRSA and HA-MRSA isolates. Six exotoxin genes were significantly more likely to be found among CA-MRSA strains and 7 were significantly more likely among HA-MRSA strains [47]. The exotoxin genes more commonly found in CA-MRSA isolates include *lukS-PV/lukF-PV* (encoding PVL), *sea, seb, sec, seh* and *sek*. The role of these toxin genes and their expressed toxins in the pathogenesis of virulent CA-MRSA infections is not well understood.

PVL is suspected to play an important role in the virulence of CA-MRSA organisms. PVL disrupts the integrity of specific cell membranes, including those of polymorphonuclear leukocytes and pneumocytes. The toxin is also presumed to cause extensive tissue damage in the lungs [48, 49]. PVL is not a newly identified virulence factor, but previously this gene was uncommonly found and seen in only about 1–2% of unselected MSSA isolates and rarely found in isolates causing bloodstream infections [47, 50, 51]. However, the *pvl* genes are commonly found among CA-MRSA isolates. *Pvl* is also commonly found in cases of severe CA-MRSA infection, such as necrotizing pneumonia and necrotizing fasciitis [52–54]. In one investigation, *pvl* presence among strains causing MRSA pneumonia was associated with higher morbidity and mortality compared to strains that lacked *pvl* [55]. However, not all models have found that *pvl* presence is a marker for more severe disease [56].

## Molecular Epidemiology of CA-MRSA

Molecular typing approaches have been used to identify and monitor the local, regional and international spread of *S. aureus* outbreak strains. Multilocus sequence typing (MLST) provides a uniform nomenclature for describing MRSA sequence types, which are assigned with reference to the MLST database (www.mlst.net) [57]. Pulsed-field gel electrophoresis is generally regarded as the most discriminating technique for strain identification. The most common strains of CA-MRSA include the

USA300 strain, which is associated with outbreaks of CA-MRSA infection in football players [58] and prisoners [59], and which is the endemic strain in the western United States [25, 60, 61]. The USA400 strain (also called the MW-2 strain) has been the cause of infection in the Midwestern United States [60, 62, 63], although the USA300 strain appears to becoming increasingly common in this region. Other strains have been found to be epidemic or endemic in Asia, Australia and Europe [13, 52, 64–66]. Interestingly, analysis of older strains of *S. aureus* suggests that CA-MRSA strains have evolved from strains (the so-called 80/81 strains) that caused pandemics worldwide in the 1950s and 1960s [13].

**Staphylococcal Chromosomal Cassette-Type Element**

In staphylococci, the *mec* A gene encodes an altered penicillin-binding protein (PBP2a) that reduces affinity to β-lactam antibiotics [67]. Molecular techniques, such as the determination of the SCC type (SCC*mec*), can sometimes help with distinction of MRSA cases that appear to be of nosocomial and community origin [61], although the use of molecular definitions to determine an isolate's origin is problematic and can be inaccurate [12]. The SCC*mec* element among CA-MRSA (type IV SCC*mec*) is often distinct from the predominant types seen among most nosocomial MRSA isolates (types I–III SCC*mec*) [67]. The SSC*mec* element in CA-MRSA strains is characterized by its smaller size and lack of genetic material conferring resistance to antibiotics other than β-lactams (types IV and V SCC*mec*) [67]. SCC*mec* IV lacks antibiotic resistance genes other than the *mecA* gene, consistent with the CA-MRSA phenotype of susceptibility to most non-β-lactam antibiotics.

There is evidence that CA-MRSA strains may be more 'fit' than the 'traditional' or HA-MRSA isolates containing SCC*mec* types II/III. Compared with MSSA strains, isolates containing SCC*mec* type II/III replicate more slowly in vitro [66]. One investigation found that CA-MRSA isolates harboring SCC*mec* type IV replicate more rapidly than these traditional HA-MRSA strains and argued that CA-MRSA may have enhanced ecologic fitness compared with SCC*mec* type II/III isolates, perhaps simply due to a shorter doubling time [66]. Another investigation reported an increased ability for CA-MRSA isolates to avoid destruction by human neutrophils and cause end-organ pathology in a mouse model [68].

**Pathogenesis of CA-MRSA Infections**

The pathogenesis of community-associated MRSA infection is incompletely understood. Models of CA-MRSA transmission have been developed to help explain factors associated with CA-MRSA acquisition. A conceptual model of CA-MRSA transmission is the 'Five Cs' model developed by the Centers for Disease Control and

**Table 1.** The 'Cs' of CA-MRSA infection

| Risk | Examples |
| --- | --- |
| Contact | direct skin-to-skin contact with infected or colonized persons |
| Cleanliness | lack of optimal personal hygiene, bathing, soap use, covering wounds |
| Compromised skin integrity | broken skin from cuts, abrasions, or dermatitis that allows MRSA to invade the skin |
| Contaminated objects, surfaces and items | fomites (such as towels, clothes, benches, etc.) that can facilitate acquisition of MRSA |
| Crowded living conditions | large number of people in a small space, which facilitates interpersonal spread of MRSA |
| Antibiotic capsules (or pills, liquids, etc.) | previous ingestion of an antibiotic by a patient, particularly ones that have activity against MSSA strains but not MRSA strains |

Adapted from references [9, 69]

Prevention (CDC) [9, 69]. This model suggests that MRSA results from a constellation of risks (table 1):

- contact
- cleanliness
- compromised skin integrity
- contaminated objects, surfaces and items
- crowded living conditions.

There are data that a sixth 'C', exposure to antibiotic capsules (and tablets, liquids, etc.), also plays an important role in MRSA acquisition [58, 70].

This conceptual model provides an important framework to study and understand MRSA infection. It is based in part on observations from outbreak investigations of MRSA risk factors conducted in well-defined populations, such football players. The validity of this framework in endemic (i.e. non-epidemic) CA-MRSA infection is less certain, although empirical data have supported several of the concepts illustrated by the model [33].

Traditionally, nasal colonization has been believed to play an important role in the development of *S. aureus* infections. The ecologic niche for *S. aureus* in humans is in the anterior nares, from which *S. aureus* can be identified most consistently in humans [71]. Although *S. aureus* can also be found on the skin of the axilla, perineum, rectum or vagina, the nose appears to be the primary reservoir for replication and spread to other bodily sites. This idea is supported by studies showing that if nasal carriage of

*S. aureus* is temporarily eliminated by use of an intranasal antibiotic, colonization often disappears from simultaneously colonized body sites [72].

The likelihood that a given person is colonized does not appear to be the same for all individuals. Studies have suggested that individuals can usually be placed into 3 groups with respect to *S. aureus* carriage: non-carriers, intermittent carriers and persistent carriers [71]. Approximately one quarter to one third of persons harbor *S. aureus* in the nose at any time [71]. Persons with underlying medical conditions such as HIV/AIDS or diabetes often have colonization rates that exceed those of the general population.

The association between *S. aureus* colonization and subsequent infection has been observed repeatedly [71, 73–75]. This relationship has been a long-held fundamental tenet in the pathogenesis of *S. aureus* infection. Nasal colonization with *S. aureus* is a risk factor for the development of clinical infection by the same *S. aureus* strain [71, 73]. More importantly, when *S. aureus* colonization is eradicated, the short-term risk of clinical infection can sometimes be lowered [71, 74, 75].

Much of the data on *S. aureus* colonization and subsequent infection may have limited relevance for CA-MRSA disease. Older investigations of colonization and disease were largely conducted in either hospital or institutional settings, such as hospital wards, nursing homes or rehabilitation units [71, 74, 75]. Non-hospitalized populations studied were almost exclusively those with heavy regular contact with the medical system and its environs, such as people on dialysis or with underlying medical conditions [76, 77]. The few data that exist on the association between nasal MRSA colonization and CA-MRSA infection suggest the relationship between colonization and infection may be less straightforward than in those found in older studies.

Several studies illustrate the role (or lack thereof) of MRSA colonization in the acquisition of CA-MRSA infection. An outbreak investigation of community-associated *S. aureus* infections in several remote Alaskan villages found that >85% of infections were caused by MRSA [78]. Among cases, controls and household contacts of cases, 40% were nasally colonized with *S. aureus*, but the majority (67%) of *S. aureus* colonization in the community was caused by MSSA. MRSA was isolated from many sauna benches in these villages. Most clinical disease occurred in the buttocks or legs, areas in contact with saunas. Not surprisingly, sauna use was a strong risk factor for infection [78]. This suggests that environmental sources may have been be an important step in the pathogenesis of infection. Alternatively, MRSA colonization may have had a higher 'attack rate' and was more likely to cause clinical infection after colonization was established.

Another investigation, of 814 US soldiers, demonstrated that only 3% were nasally colonized with MRSA and 28% were MSSA colonized [79]. However, all clinical disease in which cultures could be performed in this population were caused by MRSA. While MRSA colonization was associated with MRSA infection, over half of the clinical MRSA infections in the soldiers [7 of 11 (64%)] occurred in those who were (retrospectively) found to *not* be nasally colonized with MRSA. An investigation of MRSA infections among a Connecticut football team (10 of nearly 100 players infected), found that nasal colonization was not detected (retrospectively) in infected players and colonization may have taken a backseat to MRSA acquisition from environmental sources [80]. A cross-sectional study of *S. aureus* nasal colonization at a HIV clinic found that although the vast majority of clinical *S. aureus* infections among this population were MRSA, MRSA nasal colonization was uncommon [7 of 158 (4%)] compared to MSSA colonization [36 of 158 (23%)] [81]. The importance of fomites (inanimate objects), such as contaminated towels or razor blades, in the pathogenesis of football outbreaks further suggests that fomites may play an important role in CA-MRSA infections [58, 82]. In summary, pre-existing nasal or other body site colonization may not explain a significant amount of CA-MRSA acquisition. Prospective studies may help clarify the role of colonization in the acquisition of CA-MRSA infection.

Host defenses, such as qualitative neutrophil function, host cytokines, skin integrity and other factors, probably play important roles that are far less understood compared to pathogen-related factors [83, 84]. Clearly, phagocytic activity plays an important role in host defenses against *S. aureus*, since patients with chronic granulomatous disease have frequent *S. aureus* infections [85]. Data also indicate that type 1 immunity (activation of phagocytic defenses) is the predominant response mechanism to *S. aureus* infections [86, 87]. Nevertheless, the role of the host in susceptibility to *S. aureus* and CA-MRSA infections is extremely understudied.

## Virulence Factors

Our understanding of the virulence determinants in CA-MRSA colonization and infection is being slowly elucidated. CA-MRSA strains often carry in their genome virulence genes not found universally in *S. aureus* strains [59, 63, 88–90]. Strains also differ in the classes of accessory gene regulators *(agr, sar)*, operons that regulate virulence gene expression [91, 92]. Genetic variation among *S. aureus* strains at the core and accessory gene levels has been associated with altered pathogenic potential [63, 89]. Accessory genes encode virulence factors that are often located on mobile genetic elements such as phages and pathogenicity islands, which could help their horizontal transfer between strains [89, 93]. There is evidence that accessory genes are not distributed uniformly among strains [89, 94].

## Diagnosis

When CA-MRSA infections manifest as skin or skin structure infection [24, 28, 29, 36, 95], many patients ascribe their skin disease to a spider bite. When queried, most patients complaining of 'spider bites' admit they did not see a spider. Furthermore, many 'spider bite' infections in the United States arise in locales that are not endemic for brown recluse spiders, a species that can cause lesions that appear similar to those of CA-MRSA [96, 97]. Hence, a history of a 'spider bite' should prompt a clinician to strongly consider MRSA infection. In terms of laboratory diagnosis, *S. aureus* is a robust organism and MRSA is typically easily identifiable with standard techniques used in clinical microbiology laboratories.


## Treatment

Treatment of CA-MRSA infection remains somewhat controversial. Vancomycin has long been considered the treatment of choice for MRSA infection because, until recently, there were no good alternatives [44, 98]. The susceptibility of CA-MRSA strains to older oral antibiotics, such as clindamycin, trimethoprim-sulfamethoxazole (TMP-SMX) and tetracyclines, has opened the door to using these agents for the treatment of CA-MRSA. Many recommend these older agents for treatment, although their efficacy in CA-MRSA treatment is understudied [37, 46, 99].

For suppurative skin infections caused by CA-MRSA and *S. aureus*, incision and drainage is a key component of therapy. Many have emphasized that antibiotic therapy may not be needed in all cases of skin infection when adequate surgical drainage can be achieved. A small randomized clinical trial showed that among patients with limited *S. aureus* skin infection who underwent surgical drainage, cure rates among antibiotic-treated and placebo-treated groups were similar [100]. Other newer studies show cure rates are high (90.5%) among patients undergoing incision and drainage when treated with placebo [101] and similar to that of active therapy [102]. Nevertheless, when incision and drainage are used without antibiotics or when inappropriate antibiotics are prescribed, failures do sometimes occur [103, 104]. Furthermore, the population in which antibiotics can safely be withheld has not been clearly defined. If antibiotics are prescribed, then empirical choices should be made with an awareness of the likelihood of a *S. aureus* infection being caused by MRSA. Additionally, local patterns of antibiotic susceptibility among CA-MRSA should be used to help direct empirical therapy against this pathogen. Susceptibility of CA-MRSA strains from several investigations are noted in table 2.

The glycopeptide vancomycin is the traditional treatment of choice for MRSA. However, it has limitations. It lacks an oral form that has systemic absorption, making it a poor candidate to treat infections in ambulatory patients. Additionally, vancomycin has been associated with poorer clinical responses compared to $\beta$-lactams for serious *S. aureus* infections [46]. The recent emergence of *S. aureus* that is resistant and or only intermediately susceptible to vancomycin is also of concern, as heavy vancomycin use may drive the emergence of these strains and hence further limit the utility of this antibiotic [46]. Finally, the optimal dosing of vancomycin still remains to be defined. Many recommend that serious MRSA infections require

**Table 2.** In vitro susceptibility of CA-MRSA strains to various antimicrobial agents: summary of results from 5 investigations

|  | Atlanta [35] | Baltimore [35] | Minneapolis [35] | Los Angeles [28] | Oakland [118] | Taiwan [141] |
|---|---|---|---|---|---|---|
| β-lactams (penicilllins and cephalosporins) | 0 | 0 | 0 | 0 | 0 | 0 |
| Erythromycin | 11 | 12 | 47 | 7 | 4 | 6 |
| Ciprofloxacin | 63 | 19 | 80 | 15 | N/A | N/A |
| Levofloxacin | N/A | N/A | N/A | 88 | 57 | N/A |
| Clindamycin[a] | 87 | 85 | 88 | 95 | 97 | 7 |
| Tetracycline[b] | 89 | 61 | 91 | 81 | 86 | N/A |
| Trimethoprim-sulfamethoxazole | 97 | 83 | 99 | 100 | 100 | 91 |
| Vancomycin | 100 | 99 | 100 | 100 | 100 | 100 |
| Newer agents against Gram-positive bacteria[c] | 100 | 100 | N/A | 100 | N/A | N/A |

Data are percentages. N/A = Not available or not reported.
[a] Does not include resistance conferred by inducible resistance (see text for details).
[b] Some tetracycine-resistant strains are susceptible to doxycline and minocycline.
[c] Including linezolid, quinopristin/dalfopristin and daptomycin. Not all strains were tested against all 3 antibiotics.

dosages that exceed traditional recommendations and serum trough targets should be 15–20 µg/ml rather than the lower targets recommended in the past [105].

In terms of older oral agents, TMP-SMX is active in vitro against most (>95%) CA-MRSA strains [27, 28, 35]. However, data on clinical efficacy are limited. The largest published trial on the use of TMP-SMX for *S. aureus* is a randomized clinical trial conducted among drug users with serious *S. aureus* infections, many of whom were bacteremic. TMP-SMX demonstrated a lower clinical cure rate for *S. aureus* infection compared with vancomycin (85 vs. 98%) [106]. TMP-SMX may be adequate therapy for less severe skin and soft tissue infections [37, 43, 46, 107], but suitable clinical trials are lacking.

Clindamycin has been used successfully to treat CA-MRSA infections [108, 109]. but resistance to this agent is more common than to TMP-SMX and is greater than 10% in some areas [35]. In a Taiwanese study, resistance to clindamycin was found to be 93% among CA-MRSA [110]. Inducible clindamycin resistance may also be a concern, although clinical data regarding the effect of clindamycin resistance on clinical outcome are extremely limited. Inducible clindamycin resistance may be seen in

MRSA isolates reported as clindamycin-susceptible but erythromycin-resistant. Some (but not all) of these isolates can develop resistance when exposed to lincosamides (such as clindamycin), macrolides (such as erythromycin) and streptogramins (such as quinopristin/dalfopristin). This inducible resistance can be detected via the use of the D-test, which when positive is considered to be diagnostic for inducible resistance [111], although the clinical significance of this finding is debatable, especially for less severe infections [108]. The ability of clindamycin to inhibit *pvl* expression is a theoretic advantage of this clindamycin [112], although the clinical benefit of this inhibition is not well delineated in the treatment of CA-MRSA.

Several tetracyclines are active against MRSA. In order of increasing in vitro activity, they include tetracycline, doxycycline and minocycline [113]. Some tetracycline-resistant strains are susceptible to doxycycline and minocycline [113]. Some doxycycline and minocycline susceptible isolates carry inducible efflux genes against tetracyclines, which may limit their clinical efficacy [114, 115]. Nevertheless, doxycycline and minocycline have been successfully used to treat MRSA infections in small case series [116]. Tigecyline is a newer minocycline derivative with good and reliable activity against MRSA [117]. There is limited experience with this agent in treatment against CA-MRSA strains. Its relatively high cost compared to older tetracyclines and lack of an oral formulation limit its utility for treatment of CA-MRSA infection.

Fluoroquinolones are not reliably active against CA-MRSA strains. In many locales, insusceptibility to fluoroquinolones among CA-MRSA has approached or exceeded 50% [28, 35, 118]. Thus, these agents are probably not useful unless the organism is known to be susceptible to earlier generation fluoroquinolones, including ciprofloxacin (susceptibility to ciprofloxacin indicates that low level or partial fluoroquinolone resistance is probably not present). Among commercially available agents, moxifloxacin and gemifloxacin have the best in vitro activity against S. *aureus*, but clinical data on the use of these agents for the treatment of CA-MRSA infection are few. Anecdotal evidence is not promising [119].

Several relatively new antimicrobials may also have limited roles in the treatment of CA-MRSA. The limitation of the newer antibiotics is that they are much more expensive than older oral agents. Additionally, heavy use of newer agents is likely to be associated with the emergence of strains resistant to the newer agents and their new antibiotic classes. Linezolid, an oxazolidinone antibiotic, comes in oral and intravenous formulation. Like clindamycin, linezolid inhibits the production of the purported MRSA virulence factor, PVL [112]. Linezolid is effective in the treatment of skin infections, pneumonia and other syndromes associated with CA-MRSA [120]. A retrospective subgroup analyses of patients from clinical trials with healthcare-associated MRSA and ventilator-associated pneumonia, linezolid has been found to be associated with higher cure rates and lower mortality compared with vancomycin [121, 122]. These analyses have been criticized for their retrospective methods and use of subgroup analyses. Thus, caution has been expressed about the risk of over-interpreting these findings [123]. Because the mechanism of action of linezolid is bacteriostatic against *S. aureus*, linezolid may not be an appropriate choice when other options exist for infections where bacteriostatic activity may be critical, such as endocarditis [46, 124].

Quinupristin/dalfopristin is another newer agent with activity against MRSA, but its use has been limited due to concerns over efficacy, poorer activity in the presence of constitutive expression of macrolide-lincosamide-streptogramin resistance found in some MRSA strains, and its requirement to be given intravenously via a central line (to decrease infusion-related adverse events) [46, 125, 126].

Daptomycin is a lipopeptide with bactericidal activity against *S. aureus* and has been approved for treatment of complicated skin and soft tissue infections caused by susceptible Gram-positive pathogens [46, 127]. The agent has impressive in vitro activity against high inoculums of S. *aureus* [128], although the clinical advantage of this activity is not well delineated. Daptomycin should not be used in the treatment of pneumonia, as pulmonary surfactant inactivates this agent and it has been found to be inferior to comparators in clinical investigations of pneumonia [129]. However, daptomycin is efficacious in the treatment of bloodstream infections and right-sided endocarditis caused by *S. aureus* [130].

There is some evidence that rifampin may provide additional benefit to standard therapy in the treatment of *S. aureus*, but the data are inconsistent and rifampin is associated with many drug interactions [131]. Thus, its use for less severe infections is probably unwarranted and rifampin should never be used as a sole agent [99]. Emerging therapies include glycopeptides with longer half lives, such as dalbavancin, oritovancin, and telavancin [132–134]. Cephalosporins and carbapenems with activity against MRSA are also in development [133, 135, 136]. Even if these drugs are approved for use, their role in the treatment of MRSA and CA-MRSA remains to be defined.

So, how is one to make sense of this confusing array of choices for the treatment of suspected or diagnosed CA-MRSA infection? The answer is not straightforward, but several clinically relevant truisms should be emphasized. First, MRSA should be considered in the differential diagnosis of any skin infection that is compatible with *S. aureus* infections, such as skin abscesses [99]. MRSA should also be considered when other syndromes compatible with *S. aureus* infection are present, such as sepsis syndrome, osteomyelitis, septic arthritis and severe pneumonia or pneumonia following an influenza-like illness, as well as new manifestations of CA-MRSA described above [99]. Second, for skin infections, incision and drainage remains the cornerstone of therapy. Antimicrobial therapy is critical, although it may be deferred in selected patients who successfully undergo incision and drainage, have very limited disease, do not have infections in body parts where poorly controlled infections have a potential to cause serious sequalae (e.g. hands, feet, face), and are not immunocompromised or at the extremes of age [99]. Specific criteria to withhold antibiotic therapy are not well defined [103]. Third, because antibiotic susceptibility cannot be predicted with 100% reliability, it is prudent to culture all patients with abscesses or purulent skin lesions

[99]. Fourth, for less severe infections that can be treated on an outpatient basis, older generic antibiotics, such as clindamycin, TMP-SMX, or a long-acting tetracycline (e.g. doxycycline or minocycline) are reasonable therapeutic approaches. For more severe infections, vancomycin, linezolid or daptomycin are warranted until MRSA susceptibilities are known and the patient has improved, although the limitations of each of these antibiotics in the treatment of certain syndromes should be well understood. Rifampin might have an adjunctive role in the treatment of severely ill patients. Most importantly, whichever agent is chosen, follow-up of MRSA susceptibilities is critical, and if the patient is infected by an organism resistant to the prescribed antibiotic, therapy needs to be reconsidered. Finally, empirical therapy against suspected community-associated *S. aureus* and MRSA infections should be based on knowledge of local susceptibility patterns of MRSA strains.

**Prevention**

Because of the large number of recurrent CA-MRSA infections and back-and-forth transmission of CA-MRSA infections among household members, clinicians are often pressed to prevent infections by eradicating MRSA body colonization [37]. A CDC report concluded that there remains insufficient evidence to warrant recommendation of routine decolonization of MRSA among patients with a single or recurrent CA-MRSA infections because there are no data evaluating this approach [99]. Despite the lack of data on the association between MRSA colonization and CA-MRSA infection, many authorities suggest considering use of a decolonization regimen as a means to prevent recurrent MRSA infection in selected situations [37, 137, 138]. Regimens include topical nasal antibiotics (such as mupirocin) to eradicate nasal colonization and/or body washes with agents such as chlorhexidine, hexachlorophene and dilute bleach solutions, to eradicate skin colonization. These recommendations exist because management of recurrent CA-MRSA infections is challenging, and patients and providers are often desperate and willing to try unproven methods to prevent future disease.

Although in health care facilities, guidelines for patients with MRSA infection or colonization exist (i.e. patients are placed under contact precautions, with visitors having to wear single-use gowns and gloves when entering the room) [6, 139], those for prevention of MRSA transmission among outpatients are relatively undeveloped. Clearly, any open wound needs to be covered with dressings and persons who come in contact with drainage from infected persons need to wash their hands carefully [99]. Guidelines for the prevention of CA-MRSA infection among members of competitive sports teams have been developed and recommend that athletes and others in close contact with each other should avoid sharing equipment and towels [140]. Additionally, common surfaces such as benches that could become contaminated with MRSA or MSSA should be carefully cleaned on a regular basis [140].

Individuals with potentially infectious skin lesions should be excluded from practice and competitions until the lesions have healed or are covered. Good hygiene, such as frequent showering and use of soap and hot water, should be encouraged among athletes, military recruits, prisoners and others who live or work in close contact with each other [140].

## References


1 Diekema DJ, Pfaller MA, Schmitz FJ, et al: Survey of infections due to *Staphylococcus* species: frequency of occurrence and antimicrobial susceptibility of isolates collected in the United States, Canada, Latin America, Europe, and the Western Pacific region for the SENTRY Antimicrobial Surveillance Program, 1997–1999. Clin Infect Dis 2001;32(suppl 2):S114–S132.

2 Brook I, Frazier EH: Clinical features and aerobic and anaerobic microbiological characteristics of cellulitis. Arch Surg 1995;130:786–792.

3 Hoen B, Alla F, Selton-Suty C, et al: Changing profile of infective endocarditis: results of a 1-year survey in France. JAMA 2002;288:75–81.

4 Javaloyas M, Garcia-Somoza D, Gudiol F: Epidemiology and prognosis of bacteremia: a 10-y study in a community hospital. Scand J Infect Dis 2002;34:436–441.

5 Weinstein MP, Towns ML, Quartey SM, et al: The clinical significance of positive blood cultures in the 1990s: a prospective comprehensive evaluation of the microbiology, epidemiology, and outcome of bacteremia and fungemia in adults. Clin Infect Dis 1997;24:584–602.

6 Mulligan ME, Murray-Leisure KA, Ribner BS, et al: Methicillin-resistant *Staphylococcus aureus*: a consensus review of the microbiology, pathogenesis, and epidemiology with implications for prevention and management. Am J Med 1993;94:313–328.

7 Washoe County District Health Department: Community-associated MRSA infection surveillance in Washoe County: final report for health care providers. Epi-News 2005;25:1–6.

8 Salgado CD, Farr BM, Calfee DP: Community-acquired methicillin-resistant *Staphylococcus aureus*: a meta-analysis of prevalence and risk factors. Clin Infect Dis 2003;36:131–139.

9 Minnesota Department of Health: Community-associated methicillin-resistant *Staphylococcus aureus* in Minnesota. Minnesota Department of Health Disease Control Newsletter 2004;32:61–72.

10 Seybold U, Kourbatova EV, Johnson JG, et al: Emergence of community-associated methicillin-resistant *Staphylococcus aureus* USA300 genotype as a major cause of health care-associated blood stream infections. Clin Infect Dis 2006;42:647–656.

11 Healy CM, Hulten KG, Palazzi DL, Campbell JR, Baker CJ: Emergence of new strains of methicillin-resistant *Staphylococcus aureus* in a neonatal intensive care unit. Clin Infect Dis 2004;39:1460–1466.

12 Maree C, Daum RS, Boyle-Vavra S, Matayoshi K, Miller LG: Community-associated methicillin-resistant *Staphylococcus aureus* strains causing health-care-associated infections. Emerg Infect Dis 2007; 13:236–242.

13 Robinson DA, Kearns AM, Holmes A, et al: Re-emergence of early pandemic *Staphylococcus aureus* as a community-acquired methicillin-resistant clone. Lancet 2005;365:1256–1258.

14 Folden DV, Machayya JA, Sahmoun AE, et al: Estimating the proportion of community-associated methicillin-resistant *Staphylococcus aureus*: two definitions used in the USA yield dramatically different estimates. J Hosp Infect 2005;60:329–332.

15 Groom AV, Wolsey DH, Naimi TS, et al: Community-acquired methicillin-resistant *Staphylococcus aureus* in a rural American Indian community. JAMA 2001;286:1201–1205.

16 Herold BC, Immergluck LC, Maranan MC, et al: Community-acquired methicillin-resistant *Staphylococcus aureus* in children with no identified predisposing risk. JAMA 1998;279:593–598.

17 Fergie JE, Purcell K: Community-acquired methicillin-resistant *Staphylococcus aureus* infections in south Texas children. Pediatr Infect Dis J 2001;20: 860–863.

18 Outbreaks of community-associated methicillin-resistant *Staphylococcus aureus* skin infections: Los Angeles County, California, 2002–2003. MMWR Morb Mortal Wkly Rep 2003;52:88.

19 Methicillin-resistant *Staphylococcus aureus* infections in correctional facilities: Georgia, California, and Texas, 2001–2003. MMWR Morb Mortal Wkly Rep 2003;52:992–996.

20 Lindenmayer JM, Schoenfeld S, O'Grady R, Carney JK: Methicillin-resistant *Staphylococcus aureus* in a high school wrestling team and the surrounding community. Arch Intern Med 1998;158:895–899.

21  Zinderman CE, Conner B, Malakooti MA, LaMar JE, Armstrong A, Bohnker BK: Community-acquired methicillin-resistant *Staphylococcus aureus* among military recruits. Emerg Infect Dis 2004;10: 941–944.

22  LaMar JE, Carr RB, Zinderman C, McDonald K: Sentinel cases of community-acquired methicillin-resistant *Staphylococcus aureus* onboard a naval ship. Mil Med 2003;168:135–138.

23  Lee NE, Taylor MM, Bancroft E, et al: Risk factors for community-associated methicillin-resistant *Staphylococcus aureus* skin infections among HIV-positive men who have sex with men. Clin Infect Dis 2005;40:1529–1534.

24  Mathews WC, Caperna J, Barber E, et al: Incidence of and risk factors for clinically significant MRSA infection in a cohort of HIV infected adults. J Acquir Immune Defic Syndr 2005;40:155–160.

25  Pan ES, Diep BA, Charlebois ED, et al: Population dynamics of nasal strains of methicillin-resistant *Staphylococcus aureus* and their relation to community-associated disease activity. J Infect Dis 2005;192: 811–818.

26  Miller LG, Diep BA: Colonization, fomites, and virulence: rethinking the pathogenesis of community-associated methicillin-resistant *Staphylococcus aureus* infection. Clin Infect Dis 2008;46:742–50.

27  Moran GJ, Krishnadasan A, Gorwitz RJ, et al: Methicillin-resistant *S. aureus* infections among patients in the emergency department. N Engl J Med 2006;355:666–674.

28  Miller LG, Perdreau-Remington F, Bayer AS, et al: Clinical and epidemiologic characteristics cannot distinguish community-associated methicillin-resistant *Staphylococcus aureus* infection from methicillin-susceptible S. aureus infection: a prospective investigation. Clin Infect Dis 2007;44:471–482.

29  Sattler CA, Mason EO Jr., Kaplan SL: Prospective comparison of risk factors and demographic and clinical characteristics of community-acquired, methicillin-resistant versus methicillin-susceptible *Staphylococcus aureus* infection in children. Pediatr Infect Dis J 2002;21:910–917.

30  Naimi TS, LeDell KH, Boxrud DJ, et al: Epidemiology and clonality of community-acquired methicillin-resistant *Staphylococcus aureus* in Minnesota, 1996–1998. Clin Infect Dis 2001;33:990–996.

31  Adcock PM, Pastor P, Medley F, Patterson JE, Murphy TV: Methicillin-resistant *Staphylococcus aureus* in two child care centers. J Infect Dis 1998; 178:577–580.

32  Charlebois ED, Perdreau-Remington F, Kreiswirth B, et al: Origins of community strains of methicillin-resistant *Staphylococcus aureus*. Clin Infect Dis 2004;39:47–54.

33  Miller LG, Matayoshi K, Spellberg B, et al: A prospective investigation of community-acquired methicillin resistant *Staphylococcus aureus* (CA-MRSA) risk factors in infected and non-infected patients (abstract 1058). 43rd Ann Meet Infect Dis Soc Am, San Francisco, 2005.

34  Young DM, Harris HW, Charlebois ED, et al: An epidemic of methicillin-resistant *Staphylococcus aureus* soft tissue infections among medically underserved patients. Arch Surg 2004;139:947–951; discussion 51–53.

35  Fridkin SK, Hageman JC, Morrison M, et al: Methicillin-resistant *Staphylococcus aureus* disease in three communities. N Engl J Med 2005;352:1436–1444.

36  Eady EA, Cove JH: Staphylococcal resistance revisited: community-acquired methicillin resistant *Staphylococcus aureus*: an emerging problem for the management of skin and soft tissue infections. Curr Opin Infect Dis 2003;16:103–124.

37  Kaplan SL: Treatment of community-associated methicillin-resistant *Staphylococcus aureus* infections. Pediatr Infect Dis J 2005;24:457–458.

38  Shay AC, Matayoshi K, Spellberg B, et al: A prospective investigation of outcomes for community-acquired methicillin resistant and susceptible *Staphylococcus aureus* infections in non-outbreak setting (abstract 1059). 43rd Ann Meet Infect Dis Soc Am. San Francisco, 2005.

39  Laibl VR, Sheffield JS, Roberts S, McIntire DD, Trevino S, Wendel GD Jr: Clinical presentation of community-acquired methicillin-resistant *Staphylococcus aureus* in pregnancy. Obstet Gynecol 2005; 106:461–465.

40  Rybak MJ, LaPlante KL: Community-associated methicillin-resistant *Staphylococcus aureus*: a review. Pharmacotherapy 2005;25:74–85.

41  Miller LG, Kaplan SL: *Staphylococcus aureus*: a community pathogen. Infect Dis Clin North Am 2009; 23:35–52.

42  Huang YC, Su LH, Lin TY: Nasal carriage of methicillin-resistant *Staphylococcus aureus* in contacts of an adolescent with community-acquired disseminated disease. Pediatr Infect Dis J 2004;23:919–922.

43  Miller LG, Quan C, Shay A, et al: A prospective investigation of outcomes after hospital discharge for endemic, community-acquired methicillin-resistant and -susceptible *Staphylococcus aureus* skin infection. Clin Infect Dis 2007;44:483–492.

44  Weber JT: Community-associated methicillin-resistant *Staphylococcus aureus*. Clin Infect Dis 2005; 41(suppl 4):S269–S272.

45  Eguia JM, Chambers HF: Community-acquired methicillin-resistant *Staphylococcus aureus*: epidemiology and potential virulence factors. Curr Infect Dis Rep 2003;5:459–466.

46 Deresinski S: Methicillin-resistant *Staphylococcus aureus*: an evolutionary, epidemiologic, and therapeutic odyssey. Clin Infect Dis 2005;40:562–573.

47 Naimi TS, LeDell KH, Como-Sabetti K, et al: Comparison of community- and health care-associated methicillin-resistant *Staphylococcus aureus* infection. JAMA 2003;290:2976–2984.

48 Lina G, Piemont Y, Godail-Gamot F, et al: Involvement of Panton-Valentine leukocidin-producing *Staphylococcus aureus* in primary skin infections and pneumonia. Clin Infect Dis 1999;29:1128–1132.

49 Boussaud V, Parrot A, Mayaud C, et al: Life-threatening hemoptysis in adults with community-acquired pneumonia due to Panton-Valentine leukocidin-secreting *Staphylococcus aureus*. Intensive Care Med 2003;29:1840–1843.

50 Panton PN, Valentine FCO: Staphylococcal toxin. Lancet 1932;1:506–508.

51 Prevost G, Couppie P, Prevost P, et al: Epidemiological data on *Staphylococcus aureus* strains producing synergohymenotropic toxins. J Med Microbiol 1995;42:237–245.

52 Dufour P, Gillet Y, Bes M, et al: Community-acquired methicillin-resistant *Staphylococcus aureus* infections in France: emergence of a single clone that produces Panton-Valentine leukocidin. Clin Infect Dis 2002;35:819–824.

53 Miller LG, Perdreau-Remington F, Rieg G, et al: Necrotizing fasciitis caused by community-associated methicillin-resistant *Staphylococcus aureus* in Los Angeles. N Engl J Med 2005;352:1445–1453.

54 Francis JS, Doherty MC, Lopatin U, et al: Severe community-onset pneumonia in healthy adults caused by methicillin-resistant *Staphylococcus aureus* carrying the Panton-Valentine leukocidin genes. Clin Infect Dis 2005;40:100–107.

55 Gillet Y, Issartel B, Vanhems P, et al: Association between *Staphylococcus aureus* strains carrying gene for Panton-Valentine leukocidin and highly lethal necrotising pneumonia in young immunocompetent patients. Lancet 2002;359:753–759.

56 Voyich JM, Otto M, Mathema B, et al: Is Panton-Valentine leukocidin the major virulence determinant in community-associated methicillin-resistant *Staphylococcus aureus* disease? J Infect Dis 2006;194:1761–1770.

57 Enright MC, Day NP, Davies CE, Peacock SJ, Spratt BG: Multilocus sequence typing for characterization of methicillin-resistant and methicillin-susceptible clones of *Staphylococcus aureus*. J Clin Microbiol 2000;38:1008–1015.

58 Kazakova SV, Hageman JC, Matava M, et al: A clone of methicillin-resistant *Staphylococcus aureus* among professional football players. N Engl J Med 2005;352:468–475.

59 Diep BA, Sensabaugh GF, Somboona NS, Carleton HA, Perdreau-Remington F: Widespread skin and soft-tissue infections due to two methicillin-resistant *Staphylococcus aureus* strains harboring the genes for Panton-Valentine leucocidin. J Clin Microbiol 2004;42:2080–2084.

60 McDougal LK, Steward CD, Killgore GE, Chaitram JM, McAllister SK, Tenover FC: Pulsed-field gel electrophoresis typing of oxacillin-resistant *Staphylococcus aureus* isolates from the United States: establishing a national database. J Clin Microbiol 2003;41:5113–5120.

61 Carleton HA, Diep BA, Charlebois ED, Sensabaugh GF, Perdreau-Remington F: Community-adapted methicillin-resistant *Staphylococcus aureus* (MRSA): population dynamics of an expanding community reservoir of MRSA. J Infect Dis 2004;190:1730–1738.

62 Four pediatric deaths from community-acquired methicillin-resistant *Staphylococcus aureus*: Minnesota and North Dakota, 1997–1999. MMWR Recomm Rep 1999;48:707–710.

63 Baba T, Takeuchi F, Kuroda M, et al: Genome and virulence determinants of high virulence community-acquired MRSA. Lancet 2002;359:1819–1827.

64 Adhikari RP, Cook GM, Lamont I, Lang S, Heffernan H, Smith JM: Phenotypic and molecular characterization of community occurring, Western Samoan phage pattern methicillin-resistant *Staphylococcus aureus*. J Antimicrob Chemother 2002;50:825–831.

65 Witte W, Braulke C, Cuny C, et al: Emergence of methicillin-resistant *Staphylococcus aureus* with Panton-Valentine leukocidin genes in central Europe. Eur J Clin Microbiol Infect Dis 2005;24:1–5.

66 Okuma K, Iwakawa K, Turnidge JD, et al: Dissemination of new methicillin-resistant *Staphylococcus aureus* clones in the community. J Clin Microbiol 2002;40:4289–4294.

67 Daum RS, Ito T, Hiramatsu K, et al: A novel methicillin-resistance cassette in community-acquired methicillin-resistant *Staphylococcus aureus* isolates of diverse genetic backgrounds. J Infect Dis 2002;186:1344–1347.

68 Voyich JM, Braughton KR, Sturdevant DE, et al: Insights into mechanisms used by *Staphylococcus aureus* to avoid destruction by human neutrophils. J Immunol 2005;175:3907–3919.

69 Ragan P: Community-acquired MRSA infection: an update. JAAPA 2006;19:24–29.

70 Coronado F, Nicholas JA, Wallace BJ, et al. Community-associated methicillin-resistant Staphylococcus aureus skin infections in a religious community. Epidemiol Infect 2006;135:492–501.

71 Kluytmans J, van Belkum A, Verbrugh H. Nasal carriage of Staphylococcus aureus: epidemiology, underlying mechanisms, and associated risks. Clin Microbiol Rev 1997;10:505–520.

72 Reagan DR, Doebbeling BN, Pfaller MA, et al: Elimination of coincident *Staphylococcus aureus* nasal and hand carriage with intranasal application of mupirocin calcium ointment. Ann Intern Med 1991;114:101–106.

73 von Eiff C, Becker K, Machka K, Stammer H, Peters G: Nasal carriage as a source of *Staphylococcus aureus* bacteremia. Study Group. N Engl J Med 2001;344:11–16.

74 Cederna JE, Terpenning MS, Ensberg M, Bradley SF, Kauffman CA: *Staphylococcus aureus* nasal colonization in a nursing home: eradication with mupirocin. Infect Control Hosp Epidemiol 1990;11: 13–16.

75 Darouiche R, Wright C, Hamill R, Koza M, Lewis D, Markowski J: Eradication of colonization by methicillin-resistant *Staphylococcus aureus* by using oral minocycline-rifampin and topical mupirocin. Antimicrob Agents Chemother 1991;35:1612–1615.

76 Khan IH, Catto GR: Long-term complications of dialysis: infection. Kidney Int Suppl 1993;41:S143–S148.

77 Laupland KB, Church DL, Mucenski M, Sutherland LR, Davies HD: Population-based study of the epidemiology of and the risk factors for invasive *Staphylococcus aureus* infections. J Infect Dis 2003; 187:1452–1459.

78 Baggett HC, Hennessy TW, Rudolph K, et al: Community-onset methicillin-resistant *Staphylococcus aureus* associated with antibiotic use and the cytotoxin Panton-Valentine leukocidin during a furunculosis outbreak in rural Alaska. J Infect Dis 2004;189:1565–1573.

79 Ellis MW, Hospenthal DR, Dooley DP, Gray PJ, Murray CK: Natural history of community-acquired methicillin-resistant *Staphylococcus aureus* colonization and infection in soldiers. Clin Infect Dis 2004;39:971–979.

80 Begier EM, Frenette K, Barrett NL, et al: A high-morbidity outbreak of methicillin-resistant *Staphylococcus aureus* among players on a college football team, facilitated by cosmetic body shaving and turf burns. Clin Infect Dis 2004;39:1446–1453.

81 Rieg G, Daar E, Witt M, Guerrero M, Miller L: Community-acquired methicillin resistant *Staphylococcus aureus* colonization among HIV-infected men who have sex with men: a point prevalence survey(abstract 877). 12th Conference on Retroviruses and Opportunistic Infections, Boston, 2005.

82 Nguyen DM, Mascola L, Brancoft E: Recurring methicillin-resistant *Staphylococcus aureus* infections in a football team. Emerg Infect Dis 2005;11: 526–532.

83 Lowy FD: *Staphylococcus aureus* infections. N Engl J Med 1998;339:520–532.

84 Waldvogel F: *Staphyloccus aureus* (including toxic shock syndrome); in Mandell GL, Bennett JE, Dolin R (eds): Mandell, Douglas, and Bennett's Principles and Practice of Infectious Diseases, ed 5. Philadelphia, Churchill Livingstone, 2000, pp 2072–2083.

85 Liese J, Kloos S, Jendrossek V, et al: Long-term follow-up and outcome of 39 patients with chronic granulomatous disease. J Pediatr 2000;137:687–693.

86 Guillen C, McInnes IB, Vaughan DM, et al: Enhanced Th1 response to *Staphylococcus aureus* infection in human lactoferrin-transgenic mice. J Immunol 2002;168:3950–3957.

87 Spellberg B, Edwards JE Jr: Type 1/Type 2 immunity in infectious diseases. Clin Infect Dis 2001;32:76–102.

88 Peacock SJ, Moore CE, Justice A, et al: Virulent combinations of adhesin and toxin genes in natural populations of *Staphylococcus aureus*. Infect Immun 2002;70:4987–4996.

89 Kuroda M, Ohta T, Uchiyama I, et al: Whole genome sequencing of meticillin-resistant *Staphylococcus aureus*. Lancet 2001;357:1225–1240.

90 Holden MT, Feil EJ, Lindsay JA, et al: Complete genomes of two clinical *Staphylococcus aureus* strains: evidence for the rapid evolution of virulence and drug resistance. Proc Natl Acad Sci USA 2004;101:9786–9791.

91 Chien Y, Cheung AL: Molecular interactions between two global regulators, *sar* and *agr*, in *Staphylococcus aureus*. J Biol Chem 1998;273:2645–2652.

92 Sabersheikh S, Saunders NA: Quantification of virulence-associated gene transcripts in epidemic methicillin resistant *Staphylococcus aureus* by real-time PCR. Mol Cell Probes 2004;18:23–31.

93 Robinson DA, Enright MC: Evolution of *Staphylococcus aureus* by large chromosomal replacements. J Bacteriol 2004;186:1060–1064.

94 Jarraud S, Mougel C, Thioulouse J, et al: Relationships between *Staphylococcus aureus* genetic background, virulence factors, *agr* groups (alleles), and human disease. Infect Immun 2002;70:631–41.

95 Huang H, C. M, Flynn N, et al: Injection drug user (IDU) and community associated methicillin-resistant *Staphylococcus aureus* (CA-MRSA) infection in Sacramento (abstract). 43rd Ann Meet Infect Dis Soc Am, San Francisco, 2005.

96 Vetter RS, Cushing PE, Crawford RL, Royce LA: Diagnoses of brown recluse spider bites (loxoscelism) greatly outnumber actual verifications of the spider in four western American states. Toxicon 2003;42:413–418.

97 Miller LG, Spellberg B: Spider bites and infections caused by community-associated methicillin-resistant *Staphylococcus aureus*. Surg Infect (Larchmt) 2004;5:321–322; author reply 2.

     

98 Kollef MH, Micek ST: Methicillin-resistant *Staphylococcus aureus*: a new community-acquired pathogen? Curr Opin Infect Dis 2006;19:161–8.

99 Gorwitz RJ, Jernigan DB, Powers JH, Jernigan JA, and Participants in the CDC-Convened Experts' Meeting on Management of MRSA in the Community: Strategies for clinical management of MRSA in the community: summary of an experts' meeting convened by the Centers for Disease Control and Prevention. 2006. Available at http://cdc.gov/ncidod/dhqp/pdf/ar/CAMRSA_Exp MtgStrategies.pdf (accessed May 22, 2006).

100 Llera JL, Levy RC: Treatment of cutaneous abscess: a double-blind clinical study. Ann Emerg Med 1985; 14:15–19.

101 Rajendran PM, Young D, Maurer T, et al: Randomized, double-blind, placebo-controlled trial of cephalexin for treatment of uncomplicated skin abscesses in a population at risk for community-acquired methicillin-resistant *Staphylococcus aureus* infection. Antimicrob Agents Chemother 2007;51: 4044–4048.

102 Duong M, Markwell S, Peter J, Barenkamp S: Randomized, controlled trial of antibiotics in the management of community-acquired skin abscesses in the pediatric patient. Ann Emerg Med 2009, E-pub ahead of print.

103 Miller LG, Spellberg B: Treatment of community-associated methicillin-resistant *Staphylococcus aureus* skin and soft tissue infections with drainage but no antibiotic therapy. Pediatr Infect Dis J 2004;23:795; author reply 6.

104 Yeh J: The role of antibiotics in community-acquired MRSA cutaneous abscesses. Infect Med 2006;23: 166–167.

105 Rybak M, Lomaestro B, Rotschafer JC, et al: Therapeutic monitoring of vancomycin in adult patients: a consensus review of the American Society of Health-System Pharmacists, the Infectious Diseases Society of America, and the Society of Infectious Diseases Pharmacists. Am J Health Syst Pharm 2009;66:82–98.

106 Markowitz N, Quinn EL, Saravolatz LD: Trimethoprim-sulfamethoxazole compared with vancomycin for the treatment of *Staphylococcus aureus* infection. Ann Intern Med 1992;117:390–398.

107 Adra M, Lawrence KR. Trimethoprim/sulfamethoxazole for treatment of severe *Staphylococcus aureus* infections. Ann Pharmacother 2004;38:338–341.

108 Frank AL, Marcinak JF, Mangat PD, et al: Clindamycin treatment of methicillin-resistant *Staphylococcus aureus* infections in children. Pediatr Infect Dis J 2002;21:530–534.

109 Martinez-Aguilar G, Avalos-Mishaan A, Hulten K, Hammerman W, Mason EO Jr, Kaplan SL: Community-acquired, methicillin-resistant and methicillin-susceptible *Staphylococcus aureus* musculoskeletal infections in children. Pediatr Infect Dis J 2004;23: 701–706.

110 Chen CJ, Huang YC, Chiu CH, Su LH, Lin TY: Clinical features and genotyping analysis of community-acquired methicillin-resistant *Staphylococcus aureus* infections in Taiwanese children. Pediatr Infect Dis J 2005;24:40–45.

111 Siberry GK, Tekle T, Carroll K, Dick J. Failure of clindamycin treatment of methicillin-resistant Staphylococcus aureus expressing inducible clindamycin resistance in vitro. Clin Infect Dis 2003;37: 1257–1260.

112 Micek ST, Dunne M, Kollef MH: Pleuropulmonary complications of Panton-Valentine leukocidin-positive community-acquired methicillin-resistant *Staphylococcus aureus*: importance of treatment with antimicrobials inhibiting exotoxin production. Chest 2005;128:2732–2738.

113 Lewis SA, Altemeier WA: Correlation of in vitro resistance of *Staphylococcus aureus* to tetracycline, doxycycline, and minocycline with in vivo use. Chemotherapy 1976;22:319–323.

114 Trzcinski K, Cooper BS, Hryniewicz W, Dowson CG: Expression of resistance to tetracyclines in strains of methicillin-resistant *Staphylococcus aureus*. J Antimicrob Chemother 2000;45:763–770.

115 Schmitz FJ, Krey A, Sadurski R, Verhoef J, Milatovic D, Fluit AC: Resistance to tetracycline and distribution of tetracycline resistance genes in European *Staphylococcus aureus* isolates. J Antimicrob Chemother 2001;47:239–240.

116 Ruhe JJ, Monson T, Bradsher RW, Menon A: Use of long-acting tetracyclines for methicillin-resistant *Staphylococcus aureus* infections: case series and review of the literature. Clin Infect Dis 2005;40:1429–1434.

117 Squires RA, Postier RG: Tigecycline for the treatment of infections due to resistant Gram-positive organisms. Expert Opin Investig Drugs 2006;15:155–162.

118 Frazee BW, Lynn J, Charlebois ED, Lambert L, Lowery D, Perdreau-Remington F: High prevalence of methicillin-resistant *Staphylococcus aureus* in emergency department skin and soft tissue infections. Ann Emerg Med 2005;45:311–320.

119 Iyer S, Jones DH: Community-acquired methicillin-resistant *Staphylococcus aureus* skin infection: a retrospective analysis of clinical presentation and treatment of a local outbreak. J Am Acad Dermatol 2004;50:854–858.

120 Moellering RC: Linezolid: the first oxazolidinone antimicrobial. Ann Intern Med 2003;138:135–142.

121 Wunderink RG, Rello J, Cammarata SK, Croos-Dabrera RV, Kollef MH: Linezolid vs vancomycin: analysis of two double-blind studies of patients with methicillin-resistant *Staphylococcus aureus* nosocomial pneumonia. Chest 2003;124:1789–1797.

122 Kollef MH, Rello J, Cammarata SK, Croos-Dabrera RV, Wunderink RG: Clinical cure and survival in Gram-positive ventilator-associated pneumonia: retrospective analysis of two double-blind studies comparing linezolid with vancomycin. Intensive Care Med 2004;30:388–394.

123 Powers JH, Ross DB, Lin D, Soreth J: Linezolid and vancomycin for methicillin-resistant *Staphylococcus aureus* nosocomial pneumonia: the subtleties of subgroup analyses. Chest 2004;126:314–315; author reply 5–6.

124 Pankey GA, Sabath LD: Clinical relevance of bacteriostatic versus bactericidal mechanisms of action in the treatment of Gram-positive bacterial infections. Clin Infect Dis 2004;38:864–870.

125 Fagon J, Patrick H, Haas DW, et al: Treatment of Gram-positive nosocomial pneumonia: prospective randomized comparison of quinupristin/dalfopristin versus vancomycin. Nosocomial Pneumonia Group. Am J Respir Crit Care Med 2000;161:753–762.

126 Livermore DM: Quinupristin/dalfopristin and linezolid: where, when, which and whether to use? J Antimicrob Chemother 2000;46:347–50.

127 Eisenstein BI. Lipopeptides, focusing on daptomycin, for the treatment of Gram-positive infections. Expert Opin Investig Drugs 2004;13:1159–1169.

128 LaPlante KL, Rybak MJ: Impact of high-inoculum *Staphylococcus aureus* on the activities of nafcillin, vancomycin, linezolid, and daptomycin, alone and in combination with gentamicin, in an in vitro pharmacodynamic model. Antimicrob Agents Chemother 2004;48:4665–4672.

129 Silverman JA, Mortin LI, Vanpraagh AD, Li T, Alder J: Inhibition of daptomycin by pulmonary surfactant: in vitro modeling and clinical impact. J Infect Dis 2005;191:2149–2152.

130 Fowler VG Jr, Boucher HW, Corey GR, et al: Daptomycin versus standard therapy for bacteremia and endocarditis caused by *Staphylococcus aureus*. N Engl J Med 2006;355:653–665.

131 Perlroth J, Kuo M, Tan J, Bayer AS, Miller LG: Adjunctive rifampin for the treatment of *Staphylococcus aureus* infections: a systematic review of the literature. Arch Intern Med 2008;168:805–819.

132 Barrett JF: Recent developments in glycopeptide antibacterials. Curr Opin Investig Drugs 2005;6: 781–790.

133 Schmidt-Ioanas M, de Roux A, Lode H: New antibiotics for the treatment of severe staphylococcal infection in the critically ill patient. Curr Opin Crit Care 2005;11:481–486.

134 Van Bambeke F: Glycopeptides in clinical development: pharmacological profile and clinical perspectives. Curr Opin Pharmacol 2004;4:471–478.

135 Guignard B, Entenza JM, Moreillon P: Beta-lactams against methicillin-resistant *Staphylococcus aureus*. Curr Opin Pharmacol 2005;5:479–489.

136 Kurazono M, Ida T, Yamada K, et al: In vitro activities of ME1036 (CP5609), a novel parenteral carbapenem, against methicillin-resistant staphylococci. Antimicrob Agents Chemother 2004;48:2831–2837.

137 Federal Bureau of Prisons: Clinical practice guidelines: management of methicillin-resistant *Staphylococcus aureus* (MRSA) infections. 2005. Available at www.bop.gov/news/PDFs/mrsa.pdf (accessed August 22, 2005).

138 Dellit T, Duchin J, Hofmann J, Gurmai Olson E: Interim Guidelines for Evaluation and Management of Community Associated Methicillin Resistant *Staphylococcus aureus* Skin and Soft Tissue Infections in Outpatient Settings. 2004. Available at www.doh.wa.gov/Topics/Antibiotics/Documents/ MRSAinterimGuidelines.pdf (accessed June 27, 2005).

139 Wenzel RP, Reagan DR, Bertino JS Jr, Baron EJ, Arias K: Methicillin-resistant *Staphylococcus aureus* outbreak: a consensus panel's definition and management guidelines. Am J Infect Control 1998;26: 102–110.

140 Methicillin-resistant *Staphylococcus aureus* infections among competitive sports participants: Colorado, Indiana, Pennsylvania, and Los Angeles County, 2000–2003. MMWR Morb Mortal Wkly Rep 2003; 52:793–795.

Loren Gregory Miller, MD, MPH
Associate Professor of Medicine, David Geffen School of Medicine at UCLA
Division of Infectious Diseases, Harbor-UCLA Medical Center
1000 W Carson St Box 466, Torrance CA 90509 (USA)
Tel. +1 310 222 5623, Fax +1 310 782 2016, E-Mail lgmiller@ucla.edu

Weber JT (ed): Antimicrobial Resistance – Beyond the Breakpoint.
Issues Infect Dis. Basel, Karger, 2010, vol 6, pp 21–34

# Infections with Organisms Producing Extended-Spectrum β-Lactamase

David L. Paterson · Yohei Doi

University of Pittsburgh School of Medicine, Suite 3A, Falk Medical Building, Pittsburgh, Pa., USA

## Abstract

Extended-spectrum β-lactamases (ESBL) are enzymes produced by a variety of Gram-negative bacilli, which confer reduced susceptibility to third-generation cephalosporins and aztreonam. Resistance to other antibiotic classes (such as aminoglycosides or fluoroquinolones) is also frequently observed in ESBL-producing organisms. Outbreaks of hospital-acquired infection with ESBL-producing organisms were recognized more than 20 years ago. Acquisition in nursing homes and other health care facilities was also noted. In more recent times, community-onset infections, sometimes in patients without health care contact, have been widely observed. The origins of community-acquired infection with ESBL-producing organisms is an area deserving much future study.



## Introduction

The discovery and subsequent development of penicillin represented a huge step forward in medicine. The development of other β-lactam antibiotics over the last 60 years has enabled physicians to treat a broad range of bacterial infections. However, the bacteria causing these infections have developed a prolific array of β-lactamases, enzymes which can lead to hydrolysis of the β-lactam ring, and therefore inactivation of the antibiotics. β-lactamases that inactivate penicillin were first described by Abraham in the 1940s. In the 1960s ampicillin was introduced into clinical practice. Within months after its release, a plasmid-mediated β-lactamase conferring resistance in *Escherichia coli* was discovered. This β-lactamase was coined the TEM β-lactamase. *Klebsiella pneumoniae* was found to be consistently ampicillin resistant. The mechanism was a chromosomally encoded β-lactamase, termed SHV.

The third-generation cephalosporins were introduced into clinical practice in the early 1980s. Shortly after their release, β-lactamases were discovered which could hydrolyze and inactivate these antibiotics. The genes encoding these β-lactamases

**Table 1.** β-lactamases which inactivate third-generation cephalosporins

| β-lactamase | Ability to hydrolyze | | |
|---|---|---|---|
| | cephamycins | cefepime | carbapenems |
| ESBLs | – | + | – |
| KPC | + | + | ++ |
| AmpC | ++ | – | – |
| MBLs | ++ | ++ | + |

were identical to TEM or SHV except for point mutations which led to an altered amino acid sequence. The subsequent structural change led to an ability to hydrolyze third-generation cephalosporins. In view of the extended spectrum of antibiotic-hydrolyzing abilities compared to the parent TEM and SHV enzymes, these β-lactamases were coined extended-spectrum β-lactamases (ESBLs). In addition to the TEM and SHV type ESBLs, many new types of ESBLs have now been described, most notably the CTX-M type ESBLs.

The ESBLs can be defined as β-lactamases capable of conferring bacterial resistance to the penicillins, first-, second- and third-generation cephalosporins and aztreonam (but not the cephamycins or carbapenems) by hydrolysis of these antibiotics, and which are inhibited by β-lactamase inhibitors such as clavulanic acid. By the classification scheme of Ambler, the ESBLs are class A enzymes [like the narrower spectrum TEM and SHV enzymes and the broader spectrum *K. pneumoniae* carbapenemase (KPC) enzymes]. The alternative classification scheme of Bush-Jacoby-Medeiros denotes ESBLs as group 2be [1]. The ESBLs are quite distinct from the AmpC β-lactamases and metallo-β-lactamases (MBLs) which also hydrolyze third-generation cephalosporins (table 1). The AmpC β-lactamases are differentiated from ESBLs by their ability to hydrolyze cephamycins. The MBLs hydrolyze carbapenems, an antibiotic class not susceptible to ESBL-mediated hydrolysis.

## Host Range and Prevalence of ESBLs

ESBLs are most frequently found in *K. pneumoniae*. ESBL-producing *K. pneumoniae* are typically hospital acquired. Hospital-acquired ESBL-producing *K. pneumoniae* have spread throughout much of the world, with highest incidences in Latin America, Asia, Turkey and parts of Eastern Europe. In a report from the National Nosocomial Infections Surveillance network of hospitals, 20.6% of *K. pneumoniae* isolates from patients in intensive care units in the United States were probable ESBL producers. There was a 47% increase in the proportion of *K. pneumoniae* isolates which were probable ESBL producers in 2003, compared to 1997–2002. *Klebsiella oxytoca* may also produce ESBLs, although the prevalence of ESBL production by this species in the United States is not known. ESBL-producing *Enterobacter cloacae* are also commonly hospital acquired. Unfortunately, laboratory detection of ESBL production by *E. cloacae* is difficult (because of the interference of the chromosomal AmpC β-lactamase in the interpretation of detection tests for ESBLs). However, hospitals which have used genetic methods for ESBL detection have found ESBLs in up to one third of *E. cloacae* isolates.

In contrast to the situation with *K. pneumoniae* and *E. cloacae*, many ESBL-producing *E. coli* are community acquired [2–9]. Typically, patients with community-acquired ESBL producing *E. coli* have urinary tract infection, and have infection with the CTX-M type of ESBLs. Some of these urinary tract infections have been associated with bacteremia. Many of these isolates are resistant to commonly used first-line agents for urinary tract infection such as trimethoprim/sulfamethoxazole and ciprofloxacin. Many reports of community-acquired ESBL-producing *E. coli* have been from Canada and Europe. In Seville (Spain), Rodriguez-Bano et al. [4] performed a case-control study examining risk factors for ESBL-producing *E. coli* infections in non-hospitalized patients and found that diabetes mellitus, prior quinolone use, recurrent urinary tract infections, prior hospital admissions and older age were independent risk factors. Pitout et al. [5], in Calgary (Canada), showed that 22.0 cases of ESBL-producing *E. coli* infection occurred per year per 100,000 population greater than 65 years of age. The cause for this sudden upsurge in community-acquired infections with ESBL-producing *E. coli* is not yet clear.

Thus far in the United States, ESBL-producing *E. coli* tend to be health care associated rather than community acquired. Nursing homes may be particularly important as sources of ESBL-producing *E. coli* in the United States. In a point prevalence study on the skilled care floor of a Chicago nursing home, 46% of residents were colonized with ESBL-producing organisms (all *E. coli*) [10]. These patients had been in the nursing home, without intercurrent hospitalization, for a mean of more than 6 months. Patients from this nursing home, as well as 7 other nursing homes, served as a reservoir for introduction of ESBL-producing organisms into an acute-care hospital [10].

A variety of other organisms have been found to produce ESBLs. Several community-acquired pathogens that commonly cause diarrhea have been found to be ESBL producers, most notably *Salmonella* [11–19]. Organisms such as *Proteus mirabilis* and *Serratia marcescens* may also produce ESBLs, although the prevalence of ESBL production by these species in the United States is not known. *Pseudomonas aeruginosa*, *Acinetobacter baumannii* and *Stenotrophomonas maltophilia* are frequently resistant to third-generation cephalosporins, but this resistance is usually caused by derepressed production of AmpC β-lactamase rather than production of ESBLs.

**Risk Factors for Colonization and Infection with Hospital-Acquired ESBL Producers**

Numerous studies have assessed risk factors for hospital-acquired colonization and infection with ESBL producing organisms [10, 20–31]. In general, patients at high risk for developing colonization or infection with ESBL-producing organisms are seriously ill patients with prolonged duration of hospital stay and in whom invasive medical devices are present (urinary catheters, endotracheal tubes, central venous lines). The median length of hospital stay prior to isolation of an ESBL-producing organism ranges from 11 to 67 days [10, 20, 21, 26, 27, 30, 32]. In addition to those already mentioned, a myriad of other risk factors have been found in individual studies, including presence of nasogastric tubes [20], gastrostomy or jejunostomy tubes [10, 25] and arterial lines [22, 23], administration of total parenteral nutrition [23], recent surgery [33], hemodialysis [26], decubitus ulcers [10] and poor nutritional status [29].

Antibiotic use is also a risk factor for acquisition of an ESBL-producing organism [23, 27, 28]. Several case-control studies have found a relationship between third-generation cephalosporin use and acquisition of an ESBL-producing strain [20, 25, 27, 28, 31, 34–40]. This is logical since organisms such as ESBL producers that are resistant to third-generation cephalosporin are likely to be selected out by use of these antibiotics. Other case-control studies have not shown an association [10, 21, 23]. A tight correlation has existed between ceftazidime use in individual wards within a hospital and prevalence of ceftazidime-resistant strains in those wards [41]. In a survey of 15 different hospitals, an association existed between cephalosporin and aztreonam usage at each hospital and the isolation rate of ESBL-producing organisms at each hospital [42, 43].

Use of a variety of other antibiotic classes has been found to be associated with subsequent infections due to ESBL-producing organisms. These include quinolones [10, 21, 27], trimethoprim-sulfamethoxazole [10, 21, 27], aminoglycosides [20, 27] and metronidazole [27]. Conversely, prior use of β-lactam/β-lactamase inhibitor combinations, penicillins or carbapenems seems not to be associated with subsequent infections with ESBL-producing organisms.

**Risk Factors for Colonization and Infection with Health Care-Associated ESBL Producers**

Within nursing homes, antibiotic use is a risk factor for colonization with ESBL-producing organisms. Antibiotic use is frequent in nursing homes; in one recent study, 38% of nursing home residents had taken a systemic antibiotic in the last month [44]. Use of third-generation cephalosporins has been identified as a predisposing event in some [45], but not all studies [10]. In contrast to the situation in acute-care hospitals, use of orally administered antibiotics (ciprofloxacin and/or trimethoprim/

sulfamethoxazole) may also be a risk for colonization with an ESBL-producing strain [10]. Nursing home residents would appear to have several additional risk factors for infection with ESBL-producing organisms: (1) they are prone to exposure to the microbial flora of other residents, especially if they are incontinent and require frequent contact with health care providers; (2) low rates of hand washing have been well documented among nursing home personnel [46]; (3) urinary catheterization and decubitus ulcers are frequent among residents [44] and have been associated with colonization of non-ESBL-producing, antibiotic-resistant Gram-negative bacilli [47, 48].

**Infection Control and ESBL-Producing Organisms**

Present evidence suggests that transient carriage on the hands of health care workers is the most important means of transfer of ESBL-producing organisms from patient to patient. Hand carriage has been documented by most [49–51], but not all investigators [52, 53], who have examined it. In these instances, the hand isolates were genotypically identical to isolates which caused infection in patients. The hands of health care workers are presumably colonized by contact with the skin of patients whose skin has already been colonized by organism [54]. Recognizing that many patients may have asymptomatic colonization with ESBL-producing organisms without signs of overt infection is important. These patients represent a significant reservoir of organisms. For every patient with clinically significant infection with an ESBL-producing organism, at least 1 other patient exists in the same unit with gastrointestinal tract colonization with an ESBL producer [22, 55]. In some intensive care and transplantation units, 30–70% of patients have gastrointestinal tract colonization with ESBL producers at any one time [23, 56, 57].

Hand carriage by health care workers is usually eliminated by hand hygiene with chlorhexidine or alcohol-based antiseptics. Several studies have documented that introduction of contact isolation precautions can lead to reduction in horizontal spread of ESBL-producing organisms. However, compliance with these precautions needs to be high in order to ensure the effectiveness of these precautions. Furthermore, we recommend that, in outbreak situations, patients who have gastrointestinal tract colonization as well as those with frank infection should undergo contact isolation (table 2). Gastrointestinal tract colonization can be detected by using media supplemented with cefotaxime or other third-generation cephalosporins.

Standard methods of hand hygiene, screening for colonization and patient isolation may not always be effective in controlling outbreaks of ESBL-producing organisms [58]. Changes in antibiotic policy may play an important role in this setting [59]. Indeed in one highly publicized outbreak, no effort was made to change infection control procedures [41]. Instead, at this hospital, ceftazidime use decreased and piperacillin-tazobactam was introduced in the formulary. In another institution,

1.  Perform rectal swabs plated on selective media to delineate patients colonized with ESBL producers

2.  Perform molecular epidemiologic assessment of isolated strains to determine relatedness of the ESBL-producing organisms

3.  If molecular epidemiologic assessment shows multiple related strains:
    (a) evaluate for the presence of a common environmental source of infection
    (b) emphasize hand hygiene
    (c) introduce contact isolation for those patients found to be colonized or infected

4.  Reduce use of third-generation cephalosporins

Rahal et al. [60] were forced to withdraw cephalosporins as an entire class in order to exact control over endemic ESBL producers. Some authors have suggested that use of β-lactam/β-lactamase inhibitor combinations, rather than cephalosporins, as the first-line empiric therapy for infections suspected as being due to Gram-negative bacilli, may facilitate control of ESBL producers [24, 41, 61]. The mechanism by which these drugs may reduce infections with ESBL producers is not certain. However, many organisms now produce multiple β-lactamases [14, 62–64], which may reduce the effectiveness of β-lactam/β-lactamase inhibitor combinations in preventing outbreaks of ESBL producers.

Because gastrointestinal tract colonization with ESBL producers is an important source of the organisms, a number of groups have previously attempted selective digestive decontamination as a means of decolonizing patients. Selective digestive decontamination has been successfully performed using regimens comprising polymyxin, neomycin and nalidixic acid [65], colistin and tobramycin [66] or norfloxacin [67]. However, in many hospitals the majority of ESBL-producing strains are resistant to quinolones or aminoglycosides, which greatly reduces the likelihood that digestive tract decontamination would work. In one institution in which nasotracheal colonization with ESBL-producing organisms was frequent, upper airway decolonization led to management of an outbreak [68]. In general, we do not recommend that 'decolonization' regimens be used given the increasing resistance observed to quinolones and aminoglycosides.

An environmental focus of ESBL-producing organisms has occasionally been discovered to be the cause of an outbreak of ESBL producers. When they are recognized and removed or properly disinfected, their impact on arresting an outbreak of infection with a multiresistant organism can be dramatic. Several examples of such an intervention have been described in the context of controlling outbreaks of infection with ESBL-producing organisms. Gaillot et al. [69] found that gel used for ultrasonography was contaminated with ESBL-producing organisms. Replacement of this gel quickly curtailed the outbreak. Branger et al. [70] found that a poorly maintained bronchoscope was colonized with ESBL-producing organisms and could be linked to respiratory tract infections with the same strain. Bureau-Chalot et al. [71] identified blood pressure cuffs as a potential reservoir for an outbreak of ESBL-producing *A. baumannii*. Repair and proper maintenance of the bronchoscope stopped nosocomial transmission of the organism. Finally, Rogues et al. [72] found colonization of 4 of 12 glass mercury thermometers with ESBL-producing *K. pneumniae* and axillary colonization with the same strain in 2 patients. Disinfection of the thermometers curtailed the outbreak.

## Laboratory Detection of ESBL Production by Gram-Negative Bacilli

Concern over ESBL detection by clinical microbiology laboratories originated because some ESBL-producing organisms appeared 'susceptible' to cephalosporins using conventional breakpoints [susceptibility indicated by a cephalosporin minimum inhibitory concentration (MIC) of 8 μg/ml or lower], allowing the potential for discordant or inappropriate treatment with an ineffective antimicrobial drug. In a review of studies which have evaluated collections of ESBL-producing organisms using standard Clinical and Laboratory Standards Institute disk diffusion or MIC breakpoints, 13–49% of isolates were found to be cefotaxime 'susceptible', 36–79% ceftriaxone 'susceptible', 11–52% ceftazidime 'susceptible' and 10–67% aztreonam 'susceptible'. Approximately 40% tested 'susceptible' to at least 1 oxyimino β-lactam and 20% to all oxyimino β-lactams [73–79].

The failure rate when cephalosporins are inappropriately used for serious infections (bacteremia, hospital-acquired pneumonia, peritonitis) with ESBL-producing organisms is substantial, and exceeds that for organisms that do not produce ESBL. Therefore, the recommendation of the CLSI is that ESBL-producing *Klebsiellae* and *E. coli* should be reported as resistant to aztreonam and all cephalosporins (including cefepime, but with the exception of the cephamycins which are not hydrolyzed by ESBLs). In clinical practice using disk diffusion or MIC testing, screening tests are performed in order to evaluate the presence of organisms likely to harbor ESBLs. Organisms meeting the screening criteria then undergo phenotypic confirmatory testing. Phenotypic confirmation of the presence of ESBLs depends on the ability to show zone diameter or MIC differences when clavulanate is added to test cephalosporins (typically cefotaxime and ceftazidime). Most semi-automated testing methods (e.g. Vitek, Microscan and Phoenix) now have phenotypic confirmatory tests for ESBL detection.

When clinical outcome data is closely reviewed it appears that there are differences in outcome of cephalosporin treatment of ESBL producers depending on the MIC of the cephalosporin used in treatment. Specifically, the failure rate of cephalosporins exceeds 90% when the MIC of the antibiotic used in treatment is 4–8 μg/ml [37, 73, 80]. In contrast, the failure rate when MICs for the treating cephalosporin were ≤2 μg/ml is substantially lower [37, 73, 80]. This data is consistent with

1. Assess whether the patient is truly infected or is merely colonized

2. If colonized, no therapy is indicated (infection control interventions may be relevant)

3. If infected, carbapenems are the therapy of choice:
   (a) meropenem or imipenem for initial therapy of bloodstream infections, hospital-acquired pneumonia or intra-abdominal infections
   (b) ertapenem for complicated urinary tract infections, for infections managed within nursing homes, streamlined hospital therapy and parenteral outpatient therapy

4. For infected patients unable to tolerate carbapenems due to allergy or other contraindication, options include tigecycline, colistin, polymyxin B and ciprofloxacin, although each has limitations (see text)

pharmacodynamic models predicting impaired outcome when conventional doses of cephalosporins are used for therapy of organisms with MICs close to the breakpoint of 8 µg/ml, but still lying within the susceptible range. The European Committee for Antimicrobial Susceptibility Testing (EUCAST) has recognized this and altered breakpoints for cephalosporins against Enterobacteriaceae. EUCAST continues to recommend ESBL detection by clinical microbiology laboratories, given the important infection control/epidemiologic impact of ESBL-producing organisms.

**Treatment of Infection with ESBL-Producing Organisms**

In vitro, the carbapenems (including imipenem, meropenem, doripenem and ertapenem) have the most consistent activity against ESBL-producing organisms because of their stability to hydrolysis by ESBLs. Carbapenems should be regarded as the drugs of choice for serious infections with ESBL-producing organisms (table 3), on the basis of increasingly extensive positive clinical experience [31, 34, 73, 81–89]. In a sub-group analysis of patients in a randomized trial of cefepime versus imipenem for nosocomial pneumonia, clinical response for infections with ESBL-producing organisms was seen in 100% (10/10) patients treated with imipenem but only 69% (9/13) patients treated with cefepime [89]. Prospective, observational studies have shown a significantly lower mortality from carbapenem-treated bloodstream infections due to ESBL-producing *K. pneumoniae*, compared to other antibiotic classes. Although synergy has occasionally been exhibited between carbapenems and other antibiotic classes [90, 91], there is no evidence that combination therapy involving a carbapenem is superior to use of a carbapenem alone [34, 88].

The choice between the different carbapenems for serious infections with ESBL producers is difficult. Published clinical experience is greatest with imipenem and meropenem. In general, MICs are slightly lower for meropenem and doripenem than for imipenem and ertapenem, although the clinical significance of this in vitro superiority is not yet clear. Ertapenem shares the good in vitro activity of the other carbapenems, although resistance rates are slightly higher than with the other carbapenems [92]. The ability to use ertapenem once daily makes it potentially useful in serious infections with ESBL producers in nursing home residents or patients continuing parenteral therapy out of hospital.

The advent of carbapenem hydrolyzing β-lactamases such as those of the KPC type and the MBLs (e.g. IMP, VIM, SPM) threatens the future utility of the carbapenems. Tigecycline is active against most ESBL-producing strains and is stable to the effects of carbapenem-hydrolyzing β-lactamases, but caution needs to be exercised when using this antibiotic for bloodstream and urinary tract infections given the low drug concentrations at these sites. Colistin and polymyxin B also have good in vitro activity against most ESBL-, KPC- or MBL-producing strains but dosing regimens are not well-established for these antibiotics, especially in critically ill individuals with renal failure. Thus far, clinical experience with tigecycline, colistin or polymyxin B for the treatment of ESBL producers is extremely limited. Fluoroquinolones are obviously not affected by β-lactamases, but co-existence of resistance mechanisms affecting the quinolones and ESBLs are frequent. Three observational clinical studies have assessed the relative merits of quinolones and carbapenems for serious infections due to ESBL-producing organisms [85, 86, 88]. Two of these studies found that carbapenems were superior to quinolones [86, 88], whereas one of the studies found that they were equivalent in effectiveness [85]. It is possible that suboptimal dosing of quinolones in the presence of strains with elevated quinolone minimal inhibitory concentrations (yet remaining in the 'susceptible' range) may account for these differences.


**Conclusions**


ESBL-producing organisms are a premier example of the growing threat of resistance in Gram-negative bacilli. In many parts of the world, rates of infection with ESBLs are growing. Yet, at the same time, therapy for ESBL-producing organisms is being compromised by other emerging resistance mechanisms in Gram-negative bacteria. This underscores several important implications for the future. Firstly, there is a need for clinical microbiology laboratories to be able to detect these resistance mechanisms. Secondly, there is a need for studies to determine the optimal means of controlling the spread of ESBL producers. Finally, there is a growing need for drug discovery efforts so that new options for treatment of ESBL producers and other multiply resistant Gram-negative bacilli.

## References

1  Bush K, Jacoby GA, Medeiros AA: A functional classification scheme for beta-lactamases and its correlation with molecular structure. Antimicrob Agents Chemother 1995;39:1211–1233.

2  Mirelis B, Navarro F, Miro E, Mesa RJ, Coll P, Prats G: Community transmission of extended-spectrum beta-lactamase. Emerg Infect Dis. 2003;9:1024–1025.

3  Colodner R, Rock W, Chazan B, et al: Risk factors for the development of extended-spectrum beta-lactamase-producing bacteria in nonhospitalized patients. Eur J Clin Microbiol Infect Dis 2004;23:163–167.

4  Rodriguez-Bano J, Navarro MD, Romero L, et al: Epidemiology and clinical features of infections caused by extended-spectrum beta-lactamase-producing *Escherichia coli* in nonhospitalized patients. J Clin Microbiol 2004;42:1089–1094.

5  Pitout JD, Hanson ND, Church DL, Laupland KB: Population-based laboratory surveillance for *Escherichia coli*-producing extended-spectrum beta-lactamases: importance of community isolates with blaCTX-M genes. Clin Infect Dis 2004;38:1736–1741.

6  Munday CJ, Whitehead GM, Todd NJ, Campbell M, Hawkey PM: Predominance and genetic diversity of community- and hospital-acquired CTX-M extended-spectrum beta-lactamases in York, UK. J Antimicrob Chemother 2004;54:628–633.

7  Woodford N, Ward ME, Kaufmann ME, et al: Community and hospital spread of *Escherichia coli* producing CTX-M extended-spectrum beta-lactamases in the UK. J Antimicrob Chemother. 2004;54:735–743.

8  Brigante G, Luzzaro F, Perilli M, et al: Evolution of CTX-M-type beta-lactamases in isolates of *Escherichia coli* infecting hospital and community patients. Int J Antimicrob Agents. 2005;25:157–162.

9  Blomberg B, Jureen R, Manji KP, et al: High rate of fatal cases of pediatric septicemia caused by gram-negative bacteria with extended-spectrum beta-lactamases in Dar es Salaam, Tanzania. J Clin Microbiol 2005;43:745–749.

10  Wiener J, Quinn JP, Bradford PA, et al: Multiple antibiotic-resistant Klebsiella and *Escherichia coli* in nursing homes. JAMA 1999;281:517–523.

11  Pessoa-Silva CL, Toscano CM, Moreira BM, et al: Infection due to extended-spectrum beta-lactamase-producing *Salmonella enterica* subsp. *enterica* serotype infantis in a neonatal unit. J Pediatr. 2002;141:381–387.

12  Bauernfeind A, Casellas JM, Goldberg M, et al: A new plasmidic cefotaximase from patients infected with *Salmonella typhimurium*. Infection 1992;20:158–163.

13  AitMhand R, Soukri A, Moustaoui N, et al: Plasmid-mediated TEM-3 extended-spectrum beta-lactamase production in *Salmonella typhimurium* in Casablanca. J Antimicrob Chemother. 2002;49:169–172.

14  Baraniak A, Sadowy E, Hryniewicz W, Gniadkowski M: Two different extended-spectrum beta-lactamases (ESBLs) in one of the first ESBL-producing *Salmonella* isolates in Poland. J Clin Microbiol. 2002;40:1095–1097.

15  Bradford PA, Yang Y, Sahm D, Grope I, Gardovska D, Storch G: CTX-M-5, a novel cefotaxime-hydrolyzing beta-lactamase from an outbreak of *Salmonella typhimurium* in Latvia. Antimicrob Agents Chemother 1998;42:1980–1984.

16  Gazouli M, Sidorenko SV, Tzelepi E, Kozlova NS, Gladin DP, Tzouvelekis LS: A plasmid-mediated beta-lactamase conferring resistance to cefotaxime in a *Salmonella typhimurium* clone found in St Petersburg, Russia. J Antimicrob Chemother. 1998;41:119–121.

17  Issack MI, Shannon KP, Qureshi SA, French GL: Extended-spectrum beta-lactamase in *Salmonella* spp. J Hosp Infect 1995;30:319–321.

18  Morosini MI, Canton R, Martinez-Beltran J, et al: New extended-spectrum TEM-type beta-lactamase from *Salmonella enterica* subsp. *enterica* isolated in a nosocomial outbreak. Antimicrob Agents Chemother 1995;39:458–461.

19  Kruger T, Szabo D, Keddy KH, et al: Infections with nontyphoidal *Salmonella* species producing TEM-63 or a novel TEM enzyme, TEM-131, in South Africa. Antimicrob Agents Chemother 2004;48:4263–4270.

20  Asensio A, Oliver A, Gonzalez-Diego P, et al: Outbreak of a multiresistant *Klebsiella pneumoniae* strain in an intensive care unit: antibiotic use as risk factor for colonization and infection. Clin Infect Dis 2000;30:55–60.

21  De Champs C, Rouby D, Guelon D, et al: A case-control study of an outbreak of infections caused by *Klebsiella pneumoniae* strains producing CTX-1 (TEM-3) beta-lactamase. J Hosp Infect 1991;18:5–13.

22  Lucet JC, Chevret S, Decre D, et al: Outbreak of multiply resistant enterobacteriaceae in an intensive care unit: epidemiology and risk factors for acquisition. Clin Infect Dis 1996;22:430–436.

23 Pena C, Pujol M, Ricart A, et al: Risk factors for fae-cal carriage of *Klebsiella pneumoniae* producing extended spectrum beta-lactamase (ESBL-KP) in the intensive care unit. J Hosp Infect 1997;35:9–16.

24 Piroth L, Aube H, Doise JM, Vincent-Martin M: Spread of extended-spectrum beta-lactamase-pro-ducing *Klebsiella pneumoniae*: are beta-lactamase inhibitors of therapeutic value? Clin Infect Dis 1998;27:76–80.

25 Schiappa DA, Hayden MK, Matushek MG, et al: Ceftazidime-resistant *Klebsiella pneumoniae* and *Escherichia coli* bloodstream infection: a case-con-trol and molecular epidemiologic investigation. J Infect Dis 1996;174:529–536.

26 D'Agata E, Venkataraman L, DeGirolami P, Weigel L, Samore M, Tenover F: The molecular and clinical epidemiology of enterobacteriaceae-producing ext-ended-spectrum beta-lactamase in a tertiary care hospital. J Infect 1998;36:279–285.

27 Lautenbach E, Patel JB, Bilker WB, Edelstein PH, Fishman NO: Extended-spectrum beta-lactamase-producing *Escherichia coli* and *Klebsiella pneumo-niae*: risk factors for infection and impact of resistance on outcomes. Clin Infect Dis. 2001;32: 1162–1171.

28 Ariffin H, Navaratnam P, Mohamed M, et al: Ceftazidime-resistant *Klebsiella pneumoniae* blood-stream infection in children with febrile neutrope-nia. Int J Infect Dis 2000;4:21–25.

29 Mangeney N, Niel P, Paul G, et al: A 5-year epide-miological study of extended-spectrum beta-lacta-mase-producing *Klebsiella pneumoniae* isolates in a medium- and long-stay neurological unit. J Appl Microbiol 2000;88:504–511.

30 Bisson G, Fishman NO, Patel JB, Edelstein PH, Lautenbach E: Extended-spectrum beta-lactamase-producing *Escherichia coli* and *Klebsiella species*: risk factors for colonization and impact of antimi-crobial formulary interventions on colonization prevalence. Infect Control Hosp Epidemiol 2002;23: 254–260.

31 Paterson DL, Ko WC, Von Gottberg A, et al: International prospective study of *Klebsiella pneu-moniae* bacteremia: implications of extended-spec-trum beta-lactamase production in nosocomial Infections. Ann Intern Med 2004;140:26–32.

32 De Champs C, Sauvant MP, Chanal C, et al: Prospective survey of colonization and infection caused by expanded-spectrum-beta-lactamase-producing mem-bers of the family Enterobacteriaceae in an intensive care unit. J Clin Microbiol 1989;27:2887–2890.

33 de Champs C, Sirot D, Chanal C, Poupart MC, Dumas MP, Sirot J: Concomitant dissemination of three extended-spectrum beta-lactamases among different Enterobacteriaceae isolated in a French hospital. J Antimicrob Chemother 1991;27:441–457.

34 Du B, Long Y, Liu H, et al: Extended-spectrum beta-lactamase-producing *Escherichia coli* and *Klebsiella pneumoniae* bloodstream infection: risk factors and clinical outcome. Intensive Care Med. 2002;28:1718–1723.

35 Eveillard M, Schmit JL, Eb F: Antimicrobial use prior to the acquisition of multiresistant bacteria. Infect Control Hosp Epidemiol 2002;23:155–158.

36 Ho PL, Chan WM, Tsang KW, Wong SS, Young K: Bacteremia caused by *Escherichia coli* producing extended-spectrum beta-lactamase: a case-control study of risk factors and outcomes. Scand J Infect Dis 2002;34:567–573.

37 Kim YK, Pai H, Lee HJ, et al: Bloodstream infec-tions by extended-spectrum beta-lactamase-pro-ducing *Escherichia coli* and *Klebsiella pneumoniae* in children: epidemiology and clinical outcome. Anti-microb Agents Chemother 2002;46:1481–1491.

38 Kim BN, Woo JH, Kim MN, Ryu J, Kim YS: Clinical implications of extended-spectrum beta-lactamase-producing *Klebsiella pneumoniae* bacteraemia. J Hosp Infect 2002;52:99–106.

39 Pessoa-Silva CL, Meurer Moreira B, Camara Alm-eida V, et al: Extended-spectrum beta-lactamase-producing *Klebsiella pneumoniae* in a neonatal intensive care unit: risk factors for infection and colonization. J Hosp Infect. 2003;53:198–206.

40 Lee SO, Lee ES, Park SY, Kim SY, Seo YH, Cho YK: Reduced use of third-generation cephalosporins decreases the acquisition of extended-spectrum beta-lactamase-producing *Klebsiella pneumoniae*. Infect Control Hosp Epidemiol 2004;25:832–837.

41 Rice LB, Eckstein EC, DeVente J, Shlaes DM: Ceftazidime-resistant Klebsiella pneumoniae iso-lates recovered at the Cleveland Department of Veterans Affairs Medical Center. Clin Infect Dis 1996;23:118–24.

42 Saurina G, Quale JM, Manikal VM, Oydna E, Landman D: Antimicrobial resistance in Entero-bacteriaceae in Brooklyn, NY: epidemiology and relation to antibiotic usage patterns. J Antimicrob Chemother 2000;45:895–898.

43 Quale JM, Landman D, Bradford PA, et al: Molecular epidemiology of a citywide outbreak of extended-spectrum beta-lactamase-producing *Klebsiella pneu-moniae* infection. Clin Infect Dis 2002;35:834–841.

44 Smith PW, Seip CW, Schaefer SC, Bell-Dixon C: Microbiologic survey of long-term care facilities. Am J Infect Control. 2000;28:8–13.

45 Rice LB, Willey SH, Papanicolaou GA, et al: Outbreak of ceftazidime resistance caused by extended-spec-trum beta-lactamases at a Massachusetts chronic-care facility. Antimicrob Agents Chemother 1990;34:2193–2199.

46 Denman SJ, Burton JR: Fluid intake and urinary tract infection in the elderly. JAMA 1992;267:2245–2249.

47 Shlaes DM, Lehman MH, Currie-McCumber CA, Kim CH, Floyd R: Prevalence of colonization with antibiotic resistant gram-negative bacilli in a nursing home care unit: the importance of cross-colonization as documented by plasmid analysis. Infect Control. 1986;7:538–545.

48 Muder RR, Brennen C, Drenning SD, Stout JE, Wagener MM: Multiply antibiotic-resistant gram-negative bacilli in a long-term-care facility: a case-control study of patient risk factors and prior antibiotic use. Infect Control Hosp Epidemiol. 1997;18:809–813.

49 Eisen D, Russell EG, Tymms M, Roper EJ, Grayson ML, Turnidge J: Random amplified polymorphic DNA and plasmid analyses used in investigation of an outbreak of multiresistant *Klebsiella pneumoniae*. J Clin Microbiol 1995;33:713–717.

50 Hobson RP, MacKenzie FM, Gould IM: An outbreak of multiply-resistant *Klebsiella pneumoniae* in the Grampian region of Scotland. J Hosp Infect 1996;33:249–262.

51 Royle J, Halasz S, Eagles G, et al: Outbreak of extended spectrum beta lactamase producing *Klebsiella pneumoniae* in a neonatal unit. Arch Dis Child Fetal Neonatal Ed 1999;80:F64–F68.

52 Szabo D, Filetoth Z, Szentandrassy J, et al: Molecular epidemiology of a cluster of cases due to *Klebsiella pneumoniae* producing SHV-5 extended-spectrum beta-lactamase in the premature intensive care unit of a Hungarian hospital. J Clin Microbiol 1999;37:4167–4169.

53 Revathi G, Shannon KP, Stapleton PD, Jain BK, French GL: An outbreak of extended-spectrum, beta-lactamase-producing *Salmonella senftenberg* in a burns ward. J Hosp Infect 1998;40:295–302.

54 French GL, Shannon KP, Simmons N: Hospital outbreak of *Klebsiella pneumoniae* resistant to broad-spectrum cephalosporins and beta-lactam-beta-lactamase inhibitor combinations by hyperproduction of SHV-5 beta-lactamase. J Clin Microbiol 1996;34:358–363.

55 Harris AD, Nemoy L, Johnson JA, et al: Co-carriage rates of vancomycin-resistant *Enterococcus* and extended-spectrum beta-lactamase-producing bacteria among a cohort of intensive care unit patients: implications for an active surveillance program. Infect Control Hosp Epidemiol 2004;25:105–108.

56 Green M, Barbadora K: Recovery of ceftazidime-resistant *Klebsiella pneumoniae* from pediatric liver and intestinal transplant recipients. Pediatr Transplant 1998;2:224–230.

57 Soulier A, Barbut F, Ollivier JM, Petit JC, Lienhart A: Decreased transmission of Enterobacteriaceae with extended-spectrum beta-lactamases in an intensive care unit by nursing reorganization. J Hosp Infect 1995;31:89–97.

58 Macrae MB, Shannon KP, Rayner DM, Kaiser AM, Hoffman PN, French GL: A simultaneous outbreak on a neonatal unit of two strains of multiply antibiotic resistant *Klebsiella pneumoniae* controllable only by ward closure. J Hosp Infect 2001;49:183–192.

59 Safdar N, Maki DG: The commonality of risk factors for nosocomial colonization and infection with antimicrobial-resistant *Staphylococcus aureus*, *Enterococcus*, Gram-negative bacilli, *Clostridium difficile*, and *Candida*. Ann Intern Med. 2002;136(11):834–44.

60 Rahal JJ, Urban C, Horn D, et al. Class restriction of cephalosporin use to control total cephalosporin resistance in nosocomial *Klebsiella*. JAMA 1998;280:1233–1237.

61 Patterson JE, Hardin TC, Kelly CA, Garcia RC, Jorgensen JH: Association of antibiotic utilization measures and control of multiple-drug resistance in *Klebsiella pneumoniae*. Infect Control Hosp Epidemiol. 2000;21:455–458.

62 Bradford PA, Cherubin CE, Idemyor V, Rasmussen BA, Bush K: Multiply resistant *Klebsiella pneumoniae* strains from two Chicago hospitals: identification of the extended-spectrum TEM-12 and TEM-10 ceftazidime-hydrolyzing beta-lactamases in a single isolate. Antimicrob Agents Chemother 1994;38:761–766.

63 Chanawong A, M'Zali FH, Heritage J, Xiong JH, Hawkey PM: Three cefotaximases, CTX-M-9, CTX-M-13, and CTX-M-14, among Enterobacteriaceae in the People's Republic of China. Antimicrob Agents Chemother 2002;46:630–637.

64 Shen D, Winokur P, Jones RN: Characterization of extended spectrum beta-lactamase-producing *Klebsiella pneumoniae* from Beijing, China. Int J Antimicrob Agents 2001;18:185–188.

65 Brun-Buisson C, Legrand P, Rauss A, et al: Intestinal decontamination for control of nosocomial multiresistant Gram-negative bacilli: study of an outbreak in an intensive care unit. Ann Intern Med 1989;110:873–881.

66 Taylor ME, Oppenheim BA: Selective decontamination of the gastrointestinal tract as an infection control measure. J Hosp Infect 1991;17:271–278.

67 Paterson DL, Singh N, Rihs JD, Squier C, Rihs BL, Muder RR: Control of an outbreak of infection due to extended-spectrum beta-lactamase-producing *Escherichia coli* in a liver transplantation unit. Clin Infect Dis 2001;33:126–128.

68 Hollander R, Ebke M, Barck H, von Pritzbuer E: Asymptomatic carriage of *Klebsiella pneumoniae* producing extended-spectrum beta-lactamase by patients in a neurological early rehabilitation unit: management of an outbreak. J Hosp Infect 2001;48: 207–213.

69 Gaillot O, Maruejouls C, Abachin E, et al: Nosocomial outbreak of *Klebsiella pneumoniae* producing SHV-5 extended-spectrum beta-lactamase, originating from a contaminated ultrasonography coupling gel. J Clin Microbiol 1998;36:1357–1360.

70 Branger C, Bruneau B, Lesimple AL, et al: Epidemiological typing of extended-spectrum beta-lactamase-producing *Klebsiella pneumoniae* isolates responsible for five outbreaks in a university hospital. J Hosp Infect 1997;36:23–36.

71 Bureau-Chalot F, Drieux L, Pierrat-Solans C, Forte D, de Champs C, Bajolet O: Blood pressure cuffs as potential reservoirs of extended-spectrum beta-lactamase VEB-1-producing isolates of *Acinetobacter baumannii*. J Hosp Infect 2004;58:91–92.

72 Rogues AM, Boulard G, Allery A, et al: Thermometers as a vehicle for transmission of extended-spectrum-beta-lactamase producing *Klebisiella pneumoniae*. J Hosp Infect 2000;45:76–77.

73 Paterson DL, Ko WC, Von Gottberg A, et al: Outcome of cephalosporin treatment for serious infections due to apparently susceptible organisms producing extended-spectrum beta-lactamases: implications for the clinical microbiology laboratory. J Clin Microbiol. 2001;39:2206–2212.

74 Jacoby GA, Han P: Detection of extended-spectrum beta-lactamases in clinical isolates of *Klebsiella pneumoniae* and *Escherichia coli*. J Clin Microbiol. 1996;34:908–911.

75 Thomson KS, Sanders CC: Detection of extended-spectrum beta-lactamases in members of the family Enterobacteriaceae: comparison of the double-disk and three-dimensional tests. Antimicrob Agents Chemother 1992;36:1877–1882.

76 Vercauteren E, Descheemaeker P, Ieven M, Sanders CC, Goossens H: Comparison of screening methods for detection of extended-spectrum beta-lactamases and their prevalence among blood isolates of *Escherichia coli* and *Klebsiella* spp. in a Belgian teaching hospital. J Clin Microbiol 1997;35:2191–2197.

77 Coudron PE, Moland ES, Sanders CC: Occurrence and detection of extended-spectrum beta-lactamases in members of the family Enterobacteriaceae at a veterans medical center: seek and you may find. J Clin Microbiol 1997;35:2593–2597.

78 Ho PL, Chow KH, Yuen KY, Ng WS, Chau PY: Comparison of a novel, inhibitor-potentiated disc-diffusion test with other methods for the detection of extended-spectrum beta-lactamases in *Escherichia coli* and *Klebsiella pneumoniae*. J Antimicrob Chemother 1998;42:49–54.

79 Cormican MG, Marshall SA, Jones RN: Detection of extended-spectrum beta-lactamase (ESBL)-producing strains by the Etest ESBL screen. J Clin Microbiol 1996;34:1880–1884.

80 Crowley BD: Extended-spectrum beta-lactamases in blood culture isolates of *Klebsiella pneumoniae*: seek and you may find! J Antimicrob Chemother. 2001;47:728–729.

81 Paterson DL: Recommendation for treatment of severe infections caused by Enterobacteriaceae producing extended-spectrum beta-lactamases (ESBLs). Clin Microbiol Infect 2000;6:460–463.

82 Wong-Beringer A: Therapeutic challenges associated with extended-spectrum, beta-lactamase-producing *Escherichia coli* and *Klebsiella pneumoniae*. Pharmacotherapy 2001;21:583–592.

83 Wong-Beringer A, Hindler J, Loeloff M, et al: Molecular correlation for the treatment outcomes in bloodstream infections caused by *Escherichia coli* and *Klebsiella pneumoniae* with reduced susceptibility to ceftazidime. Clin Infect Dis 2002;34:135–146.

84 Meyer KS, Urban C, Eagan JA, Berger BJ, Rahal JJ: Nosocomial outbreak of *Klebsiella* infection resistant to late-generation cephalosporins. Ann Intern Med 1993;119:353–358.

85 Kang CI, Kim SH, Park WB, et al: Bloodstream infections due to extended-spectrum beta-lactamase-producing *Escherichia coli* and *Klebsiella pneumoniae*: risk factors for mortality and treatment outcome, with special emphasis on antimicrobial therapy. Antimicrob Agents Chemother 2004;48: 4574–4581.

86 Endimiani A, Luzzaro F, Perilli M, et al: Bacteremia due to *Klebsiella pneumoniae* isolates producing the TEM-52 extended-spectrum beta-lactamase: treatment outcome of patients receiving imipenem or ciprofloxacin. Clin Infect Dis 2004;38:243–251.

87 Burgess DS, Hall RG 2nd, Lewis JS 2nd, Jorgensen JH, Patterson JE: Clinical and microbiologic analysis of a hospital's extended-spectrum beta-lactamase-producing isolates over a 2-year period. Pharmacotherapy 2003;23:1232–1237.

88 Paterson DL, Ko WC, Von Gottberg A, et al: Antibiotic therapy for *Klebsiella pneumoniae* bacteremia: implications of production of extended-spectrum beta-lactamases. Clin Infect Dis 2004;39: 31–37.

89 Zanetti G, Bally F, Greub G, et al: Cefepime versus imipenem-cilastatin for treatment of nosocomial pneumonia in intensive care unit patients: a multicenter, evaluator-blind, prospective, randomized study. Antimicrob Agents Chemother 2003;47:3442–3447.

90 Roussel-Delvallez M, Sirot D, Berrouane Y, et al: Bactericidal effect of beta-lactams and amikacin alone or in association against *Klebsiella pneumoniae* producing extended spectrum beta-lactamase. J Antimicrob Chemother 1995;36:241–246.

91 Pattharachayakul S, Neuhauser MM, Quinn JP, Pendland SL: Extended-spectrum beta-lactamase (ESBL)-producing *Klebsiella pneumoniae*: activity of single versus combination agents. J Antimicrob Chemother 2003;51:737–799.

92 Jacoby G, Han P, Tran J: Comparative in vitro activities of carbapenem L-749,345 and other antimicrobials against multiresistant gram-negative clinical pathogens. Antimicrob Agents Chemother 1997;41: 1830–1831.

David L. Paterson, MD, PhD
University of Pittsburgh School of Medicine
Suite 3A, Falk Medical Building
3601 5th Avenue, Pittsburgh PA 15213 (USA)
Tel. +1 412 648 6478, Fax +1 412 648 6399, E-Mail patersond@dom.pitt.edu

Weber JT (ed): Antimicrobial Resistance – Beyond the Breakpoint.
Issues Infect Dis. Basel, Karger, 2010, vol 6, pp 35–50

# Fluoroquinolone Resistance: Challenges for Disease Control

Christopher M. Parry

School of Infection and Host Defence, Faculty of Medicine, University of Liverpool, Duncan Building,
Liverpool, UK

## Abstract

The fluoroquinolones are an effective and widely used group of antimicrobials in community- and
healthcare-associated infections, including those caused by *Salmonella enterica*, *Campylobacter* spp.,
*Escherichia coli*, *Klebsiella* spp., *Pseudomonas aeruginosa*, *Neisseria gonorrhoeae* and *Streptococcus
pneumoniae*. Decreased susceptibility and full resistance to fluoroquinolones has emerged in each
of these pathogens, causing treatment failures. The widespread use of fluoroquinolones in humans
and in animal husbandry has been an important driver of resistance. Clonal spread, in hospitals and
the community, aided by the international movement of humans and transport of food, has led to
the worldwide dissemination of resistant strains. A reassessment of fluoroquinolone breakpoints to
detect first-step resistant mechanisms, attention to dose regimens and adherence to appropriate
use in humans and in animal husbandry is essential if this valuable group of antimicrobials are to
remain useful. 

The fluoroquinolones have proved to be a successful and widely used group of antimicrobials over the last 20 years. In 2002 they were the most commonly prescribed
antimicrobial to adults in the United States, accounting for 24% of antimicrobial prescribing [1]. This pattern is of usage is mirrored in many other countries, including
developing nations [2]. Unfortunately, resistance has emerged in a variety of bacteria
and clinical failure of treatment in individual patients has been the result. Rates of
resistance vary by organism and geographical region, and in some instances resistance
threatens to curtail the future effectiveness of these agents. Understanding the drivers of resistance is important so that measures can be taken to retain the use of these
antimicrobials. This topic will be reviewed with particular attention to *Salmonella
enterica*, *Campylobacter* spp. and other Gram-negative bacilli, as well as *Neisseria gonorrhoeae* and *Streptococcus pneumoniae*.

The original quinolone antibacterial, nalidixic acid, was discovered in the early
1960s and had a narrow spectrum of activity [3]. Addition of a fluorine atom at the

**Table 1.** A classification of fluoroquinolones for use in humans

| Quinolone | Current usage |
| --- | --- |
| *First Generation* | |
| Nalidixic acid | limited |
| *Second Generation* | |
| Norfloxacin | limited |
| Ciprofloxacin | widespread |
| Ofloxacin | limited |
| Enoxacin | limited |
| Fleroxacin | limited |
| Pefloxacin | limited |
| Lomefloxacin | limited |
| *Third generation* | |
| Levofloxacin | widespread |
| Gatifloxacin | widespread in certain countries |
| Grepafloxacin | withdrawn |
| Sparfloxacin | withdrawn |
| Temafloxacin | withdrawn |
| *Fourth generation* | |
| Moxifloxacin | widespread |
| Gemifloxacin | limited |
| Trovafloxacin | withdrawn |

C-6 position and piperanzinyl or related ring at position C-7 of the quinolone molecule resulted in the fluoroquinolone group with broader activity, and these became available in the 1980s (table 1). Second-generation quinolones had high in vitro activity against Gram-negative bacteria, favorable pharmacokinetics that allowed oral administration and relative affordability. They were effective in treating a wide variety of Gram-negative infections, including gastrointestinal infections due to *S. enterica* and *Campylobacter* spp., urinary infections, hospital-acquired pneumonia and invasive infections due to *Escherichia coli*, *Klebsiella* spp. and *Pseudomonas aeruginosa*, and sexually transmitted infections, particularly *N. gonorrhoeae*. A lack of activity against Gram-positive bacteria, such as *S. pneumoniae*, and against anaerobes led to further modifications of the quinolone nucleus and the development of the newer extended spectrum third- and fourth-generation quinolones, including gatifloxacin and moxifloxacin. Later generation fluoroquinolones were licensed for treating lower respiratory tract infections that were unresponsive to first-line antimicrobials, and they are being evaluated for the treatment of tuberculosis. The most commonly used fluoroquinolones in humans are ciprofloxacin, levofloxacin, gatifloxacin and moxifloxacin [3].

## Mechanisms of Resistance

Fluoroquinolones are rapidly bactericidal and associated with a prolonged post-antibiotic effect. The principal mechanism of action for the fluoroquinolones is inhibition of the bacterial DNA gyrase, resulting in the disruption of DNA replication and cell death [3]. The targeted enzymes, DNA gyrase (topoisomerase II) and DNA topoisomerase IV cooperate in the processes of DNA replication, transcription, recombination and repair. Single point mutations leading to amino acid changes in the topisomerase enzymes can lead to a decreased affinity of the fluoroquinolones for their target, and this is the commonest mechanism by which resistance is acquired. In Gram-negative bacteria the principal target is the DNA gyrase, in particular *gyrA*, and first-step mutations confer resistance to nalidixic acid and give a ciprofloxacin minimum inhibitory concentration (MIC) for most Enterobacteriacae of 0.125–1.0 mg/1, compared to the wild type MIC ≤0.03mg/1. Further mutations in *gyrA*, *parC*, to a lesser extent in *parE* and rarely in *gyrB*, move the MIC into the non-susceptible range with MICs ≥2.0 µg/ml [4]. In Gram-positive bacteria the first-step mutantions typically occur in topoisomerase IV, particularly *parC*, with subsequent mutations in *gyrA* and *parE* [5].

Altered access of the drugs to the target is a second mechanism of quinolone resistance [4–6]. The combination of alteration in drug entry and mutations in the topoisomerase enzymes can result in full fluoroquinolone resistance with MICs ≥4 µg/ml [7]. Resistance to quinolones can also be mediated by *qnrA*, *qnrB* and *qnrS* genes, which are carried on transferable plasmids. The *qnr* genes produce the Qnr protein of the pentapeptide repeat family that protects the quinolone target from ciprofloxacin inhibition. Qnr plasmids are found in *E. coli*, *Klebsiella* spp. and *S. enterica* in North America, Europe, North Africa and Asia [8]. In addition, a variant of the aminoglycoside acetyltransferase enzyme, AAC(6′)-1b-cr, produced by a clinical isolates of *E. coli* reduces the activity of ciprofloxacin by *N*-acetylation at the amino nitrogen on its piperazinyl substituent [9]. Although the increment in MIC is small with these plasmid-carried genes, they facilitate the selection of more resistant mutants and act additively with other resistance mechanisms to produce a clinically resistant strain [10].

## Detection of Resistance in the Clinical Laboratory

Fluoroquinolone resistance may be detected in the clinical laboratory by disc susceptibility or MIC testing [11, 12]. In some bacteria the breakpoints established for this purpose by the Clinical and Laboratory Standards Institute (CLSI; formerly the National Committee on Clinical Laboratory Standards) and several other national organizations do not detect the small increases in MIC that first-step resistance mechanisms may cause. The ciprofloxacin breakpoints for Gram-negative bacteria are typically set at ≤1 µg/ml for susceptibility and ≥4 µg/ml for resistance [11]. The MIC to ciprofloxacin for many wild-type Gram-negative bacteria such as *E. coli* and

*S. enterica* is ≤0.03 µg/ml. Isolates with a single point mutation in *gyrA* typically have an MIC 0.125–1.0 µg/ml and would be classified as susceptible by the current breakpoints. The same applies for other first-step resistance mechanisms and for other bacteria, such as *S. pneumoniae* [5].

For several bacteria, such as *S. enterica*, the presence of decreased susceptibility to ciprofloxacin is clinically important. Patients with invasive infections due to these strains, particularly enteric fever, respond less well to fluoroquinolones when compared with infections due to wild-type strains [13–15]. These strains are usually resistant to nalidixic acid. In one study of 1,010 non-typhoidal *Salmonella* isolates, nalidixic acid resistance had a sensitivity of 100% and a specificity of 87% for detecting strains with a ciprofloxacin MIC ≥0.125 µg/ml [16]. Similar results have been obtained for *S. enterica* serotype Typhi [14].

Recent guidelines have suggested that decreased susceptibility to fluoroquinolones in invasive isolates of *S. enterica* should be established by nalidixic acid resistance or a ciprofloxacin MIC. However, in a report of *S. enterica* serotype Typhi isolated from patients in England, Scotland and Wales, of the 271/692 (39%) isolates with reduced fluoroquinolone susceptibility, 49 (18%) of these isolates were nalidixic acid susceptible [17]. This and other reports suggest that nalidixic acid-resistance screening does not reliably detect isolates with decreased susceptibility. In areas where enteric fever is endemic, microbiology laboratories will be unable to perform MIC testing. New disc susceptibility breakpoints that detect isolates with decreased ciprofloxacin susceptibility between 0.125 and 1.0 µg/ml are needed. In *N. gonorrhoeae* current breakpoints accommodate this issue. Decreased susceptibility to ciprofloxacin and ofloxacin is defined by the CLSI as an MIC of 0.125–0.5 and 0.5–1.0 µg/ml, respectively. An MIC of ≥1 µg/ml for ciprofloxacin and ≥2 µg/ml for ofloxacin is defined as resistant [11].


**Prevalence of Resistance in Selected Pathogens**

Enteric fever caused by invasive infection with *S. enterica* serotype Typhi and serotype Paratyphi A is associated with significant mortality unless treated with antimicrobials. It is restricted to humans and is common in many developing countries where sanitation is inadequate and clean water lacking. The many other serovars of *S. enterica* (the non-Typhi Salmonellae) typically cause self-limiting diarrhea that does not require antimicrobial therapy. Infection is commonly acquired by eating uncooked or inadequately food that is contaminated with salmonella. Poultry, eggs, pigs and cattle are common sources. The non-Typhi serovars can be invasive, with bloodstream or deep-seated infections causing life-threatening disease. The elderly, patients under immunosuppression, HIV infection and infants in sub-Saharan Africa are particularly susceptible, and antimicrobials are life saving.

Fluoroquinolones have been widely used for treating drug-resistant enteric fever and invasive salmonellosis since the late 1980s. Widespread use in humans in

**Table 2.** Quinolone resistant rates in *S. enterica* serotype Typhi and Paratyphi A

| Year | Location | Serotype | Isolates n | Nalidixic acid resistant/ reduced ciprofloxacin susceptibility, %[a] | Ciprofloxacin non-susceptible, %[b] | Ref. |
|---|---|---|---|---|---|---|
| 2004 | Kathmandu, Nepal | Typhi | 409 | 50.5 | 0.25 | [18] |
|  |  | Paratyphi A | 198 | 75.3 | 0.5 |  |
| 2000–2003 | New Dehli, India | Typhi | 472 | 66.0 | 0 | [19] |
|  |  | Paratyphi A | 90 | 80.0 | 0 |  |
| 2001–2003 | New Dehli, India | Typhi | 304 | 74.3 | 0 | [20] |
|  |  | ParatyphiA | 73 | 76.7 | 2.7 |  |
| 2000 | Mumbai, India | Typhi | 240 | 82.0 | 0 | [21] |
| 2005 | Dhaka, Bangladesh | Typhi | 428 | 90.7 | 2.3 | [22] |
| 2000–2002 | Nairobi, Kenya | Typhi | 102 | 47.1 | 0 | [23] |
| 2001 | 10 European countries | Typhi | 245 | 26.0 | 0 | [24] |
|  |  | Paratyphi A | 217 | 18.0 | 0 |  |
| 2000–2003 | England and Wales | Typhi | 692 | 39.0 | 0 | [17] |

[a] MIC 0.125–1.0 µg/ml; [b] MIC >1.0 µg/ml

developing countries and in animal husbandry worldwide, has led to the emergence of isolates of *S. enterica* with decreased susceptibility. These have reached high levels in some areas, as summarized in table 2. Resistance has also been a problem in enteric fever in immigrants and returning travelers, particularly those coming from the Indian sub-continent [17, 24]. Sporadic isolates of Typhi and Paratyphi A with full resistance to fluoroquinolones, mediated by double mutations in *gyrA* and one in *parC*, have been reported in India, Pakistan and Bangladesh [22, 25–29].

Decreased susceptibility to fluoroquinolones has also been documented in the zoonotic Salmonellas (table 3) and associated with recent foreign travel, particularly to Spain and Thailand [32, 33]. Studies have documented high rates in serovars such as Enteritidis PT 1 and PT 21, Hadar and Virchow [30, 31, 34]. Taiwan has had a particular problem with *S. enterica* serotype Choleraesuis, a serovar that can cause invasive disease [36]. In a nationwide surveillance study in 2001, full ciprofloxacin resistance was found in 2.7% of isolates, with a level of 1.4% in Typhimurium and 7.5% in Choleraesuis isolates [37]. The appearance of resistance to both ciprofloxacin and extended spectrum cephalosporins in Choleraesuis serotypes is worrying [38]. Although ciprofloxacin resistance in *S. enterica* is usually associated with between 1 and 3 mutations in *gyrA*, *parC*, *gyrB* and alterations in drug influx/efflux [39], evidence is also accruing of the occurrence of

**Table 3.** Quinolone resistant rates in non enteric fever *S. enterica* serotypes

| Year | Location | Serotype | Isolates n | Nalidixic acid resistant/ reduced ciprofloxacin susceptibility, %[a] | Ciprofloxacin non-susceptible, %[b] | Ref. |
|---|---|---|---|---|---|---|
| 2003 | United States | All | 1,865 | 2.3 | 0.1 | [30] |
| 2000 | Europe | All | 22,917 | 14.0 | 0.5 | [31] |
| | | Enteritidis | 14,636 | 13.0 | 0.4 | |
| | | Typhimurium | 6,777 | 8.0 | 0.6 | |
| | | Hadar | 622 | 57.0 | 3.0 | |
| | | Virchow | 449 | 53.0 | 0.9 | |
| 2000 | Denmark | Enteritidis | 366 | 8.5 | 0 | [32] |
| 2000–2004 | Finland | All | 1,004 | 21.3 | 0.3 | [33] |
| | | | 504 | 15.0 (domestic) | | |
| | | | 500 | 39.0 (travel related) | | |
| 2001–2003 | Spain | All | 5,777 | 35.0 | 0 | [34] |
| | | Enteritidis | 3,491 | 49.9 | 0 | |
| | | Typhimurium | 1,211 | 7.5 | 0 | |
| | | Hadar | 147 | 91.2 | 0 | |
| 2000–2002 | Korea | All | 206 | 21.8 | 0 | [35] |
| 2001 | Taiwan | All | 671 | | 2.7 | [36] |
| | | Choleraesuis | 107 | | 7.5 | |

[a] MIC 0.125–1.0 µg/ml; [b] MIC >1.0 µg/ml

plasmid mediated-quinolone resistance, sometimes linked to extended-spectrum β-lactamase (ESBL) genes [40, 41].

*Campylobacter* spp. are a common cause of gastroenteritis in most countries. They are commensal in birds, swine and cattle, and infection in humans is invariably food-associated. *Campylobacter* is intrinsically less susceptible to fluoroquinolones than *Salmonella* with a wild-type $MIC_{90}$ of 0.25 µg/ml. Single point mutations in the quinolone resistance determining regions of *gyrA* result in an MIC $\geq 2$ µg/ml, which is non-susceptible by CLSI guidelines [42]. Fluoroquinolone resistant *Campylobacter* spp. in humans and animals, first reported in the late 1980s, have been documented in numerous countries [43]. Ciprofloxacin resistance in human *Campylobacter* isolates submitted through national surveillance in the United States increased from 13% in 1997 to 19% in 2004 [44]. In the same study, ciprofloxacin-resistant *Campylobacter* was isolated from 10% of chicken products purchased in 3 states in 1999 [45].

The emergence of resistance is now limiting ciprofloxacin use in local and systemic infections with Gram-negative bacilli such as *E. coli*, *Klebsiella* and *Pseudomonas*. In

US intensive care units, the overall resistance of Gram-negative bacilli to ciprofloxacin increased from 14% in 1994 to 24% in 2000 [46]. The rates were 3% in *E. coli*, 12% in *Klebsiella pneumoniae*, 10% in *Enterobacter* spp. and 24% in *Pseudomonas aeruginosa*. In 1999 in England and Wales, blood culture isolates were found to be ciprofloxacin resistant for 3.7% of *E. coli*, 7.1% of *Klebsiella* spp. and 10.5% of *Enterobacter* spp. [47]. In a prospective study of 452 episodes of *K. pneumoniae* bacteraemia in 12 hospitals in 7 countries, 5.5% were caused by isolates that were ciprofloxacin resistant [48]. Of particular note in this study was that ESBL production was detected in 60% of the ciprofloxacin-resistant isolates compared with 16% of the ciprofloxacin-susceptible strains (p = 0.0001). A similar result was seen in a case-control study in a hospital in Philadelphia, where 43 (55.8%) of 77 ESBL-producing *E. coli* or *K. pneumoniae* were found to be fluoroquinolone resistant [49].

Antimicrobial resistance is severely hampering attempts at global control of gonorrhea [50]. Single-dose oral ciprofloxacin or ofloxacin was introduced for treating gonococcal infections at a time when resistance to penicillin, tetracyclines and spectinomycin was appearing. In South-East Asia low-level resistant strains appeared in the early 1980s and full resistance in 1991. Since then, the incidence of resistant strains in many countries in Asia and elsewhere has increased markedly [50]. More than 10,000 gonococcal isolates from 15 participating countries in the WHO Western Pacific Region were examined in 2004 as part of the GRASP study [51]. The proportion of quinolone-resistant *N. gonorrhoeae* varied from 2 per cent in New Caledonia and Papua New Guinea to nearly 100 per cent in Hong Kong and China. In Japan, South Korea, Lao People's Democratic Republic and Viet Nam levels have reached about 85%. In the United States resistance increased from <1% in 2001 to 13.3% in the first half of 2006 [52], and in 12 European countries rate was 30.9% in 2004 [53].

Resistance to β-lactam and macrolide antimicrobials in *S. pneumoniae* has led to the widespread promotion of new generation fluoroquinolones for lower respiratory tract infections. Although the overall resistance to quinolones is currently low (<5%), the incidence is increasing. In Canada, ciprofloxacin resistance increased from <1% in 1997 to 4.2% in 2005 [54]. The resistance rates to other fluoroquinolones in 2005 were 1.1% for levofloxacin, 1.6% for gatifloxacin, 1.0% for gemifloxacin and 1.0% for moxifloxacin. In a Hong Kong study of 1,388 pneumococcal isolates collected between 2000 and 2005, 10.5% were resistant to ciprofloxacin and 1.6% to levofloxacin [55]. Most fluoroquinolone resistant isolates were the Spain[23F]-1 clone, a clone that has shown its ability to spread worldwide.


**Therapeutic and Public Health Implications of Resistance**


There is good evidence that infections caused by *S. enterica* with decreased fluoroquinolone susceptibility respond less well to fluoroquinolone treatment, with a significant proportion of patients (although not all) failing therapy [13–15, 19, 20]. In south

India, 8 of 38 patients infected with nalidixic acid-resistant *S. enterica* serotype Typhi were found to have a positive blood culture after 6 days of ciprofloxacin at a dose of 500 mg orally or 400 mg intravenously twice daily [56]. In a clinical trial conducted in Viet Nam, where nalidixic acid resistance is common, only two thirds of patients with uncomplicated typhoid fever responded satisfactorily to 7 days of ofloxacin [57]. For non-typhoidal *Salmonella* much of the data is from case reports [13, 14]. In one outbreak of 25 culture-confirmed cases where the strain had decreased susceptibility to fluoroquinolones, 5 patients were treated with fluoroquinolones. Of these 5 patients, 4 failed therapy, 3 with persistent diarrhea and 1 developed an intestinal perforation [58].

Evidence also exists for treatment failure in quinolone-resistant gonoccocal infection. In a prospective study of 217 female sex workers in Dhaka, Bangladesh, 37.8% of recovered gonococcal isolates were resistant to ciprofloxacin [59]. Among the patients who had successful treatment, 95% of the isolated organisms had an MIC between 0.008 and 0.06 µg/ml. For those with unsuccessful treatment, 96% had isolates with an MIC of 1–32 µg/ml. A failure rate of 32.3% was seen in women treated with oral ciprofloxacin (500 mg) in a study in the Philippines [60]. Bacteriologically proven treatment failure occurred in 14 (46.7%) of 30 women with isolates with a ciprofloxacin MIC of ≥4 µg/ml and 1 (3.6%) of 28 infected by strains with MICs <4 µg/ml. In the United States, ciprofloxacin is no longer recommended for treating gonorrhea because of the increase in resistance levels [52]. Treatment failures have also been described in case reports of patients with respiratory tract infections due to *S. pneumoniae* treated with ciprofloxacin or levofloxacin [61, 62]. In these reports, resistance was present at the outset or emerged during the course of treatment.

Increased transmission and consequent disease outbreaks can occur when drug-resistant bacteria appear. In the first 6 months of 1997, contaminated drinking water caused an outbreak of typhoid fever in Dushanbe (Tajikistan) in which 8,901 cases were reported, with 95 associated deaths [63]. Of the isolates tested, the majority were resistant to multiple drugs, including nalidixic acid. An outbreak of *S. enterica* serotype Schwarzengrund occurred in 2 nursing homes and a hospital in the United States [64]. The index patient had been hospitalized in the Philippines and had probably acquired the infection there before transfer to the United States. Transmission occurred in the nursing homes and hospital. A hospital outbreak in Canada occurred over the course of a 20-month period in a respiratory ward where ciprofloxacin was frequently used for treating lower respiratory tract infections [65]. Sixteen patients with chronic bronchitis developed a hospital-acquired lower respiratory infection with penicillin- and ciprofloxacin- resistant *S. pneumoniae* serotype 23F. At least 5 of the patients failed ciprofloxacin therapy.

Quinolone resistance may also be associated with an increased risk of severe disease and death. In a matched cohort study, Helms et al. [66] determined the death rates associated with drug resistance in *S. enterica* serotype Typhimurium. By linking the Danish Enteric Pathogen registry with national registration systems, they compared the 2-year death rates with a matched sample of the general Danish population after adjusting for differences in comorbidity. Patients with susceptible strains of serotype Typhimurium were 2.3 times more likely to die within 2 years after infection compared with the persons in the general population. Patients infected with a strain resistant to ampicillin, chloramphenicol, streptomycin, sulphonamide and tetracycline were 4.8 times more likely to die, and those infected with a quinolone (nalidixic acid)-resistant strain were 10.3 times more likely to die compared with the general population. In a second cohort study in 1,323 patients infected with *S. enterica* serotype Typhimurium, after adjustment for age, sex and comorbidity, infection with a quinolone-resistant isolate was associated with a 3.15-fold (95% CI 1.39–7.10) higher risk of invasive illness or death within 90 days of infection compared with that observed for infection with a pan-susceptible strain [67]. It was not possible to distinguish whether a poor outcome was due to the increased virulence of resistant bacteria or because of poor response to treatment.

A further potential result of antimicrobial resistance is that of collateral damage [68]. This refers to the unwanted ecological adverse effects of antimicrobial therapy in the presence of drug resistance. Fluoroquinolone usage in hospitals may inadvertently lead to increases in other multiresistant pathogens. Fluoroquinolone usage has been an important risk factor for *Clostridium difficile*-associated diarrhea and methicillin-resistant *Staphylococcus aureus* in hospitals [69, 70]. Unrelated antimicrobial use may also lead to an increase in the number of infections due to susceptible and multiresistant *Salmonellae* by causing a transient decrease in the resistance to non-commensal bacteria and increasing the likelihood of infection upon exposure to a gastrointestinal pathogen [71]. The additional 'selective effect' of antimicrobial resistance has been calculated to result in a more than 3-fold increase in vulnerability to infection by an antimicrobial-resistant pathogen among individuals receiving antibiotics for an unrelated reason. This has been estimated to lead to 29,379 additional non-Typhi *Salmonella* infections in the USA each year, including 342 hospitalizations and 12 deaths and an additional 17,668 *Campylobacter jejuni* infections, leading to 95 hospitalizations [71].

**Drivers of Resistance**

A variety of factors are considered to drive fluoroquinolone resistance in bacteria (table 4). The key factor is that widespread usage of an antibiotic applies a selective pressure to a bacterial population, which leads to resistance. A number of studies have shown a relationship between fluoroquinolone use and resistance. In Spain between 1988 and 1992, the increase in ciprofloxacin resistance in *E. coli* isolates causing bacteremia correlated with an increasing use of ciprofloxacin in the community and in hospitals and prior fluoroquinolone use was an independent risk factor for ciprofloxacin resistant *E. coli* bacteremia [72]. In the 1990s, use of fluoroquinolones in

**Table 4.** Drivers of fluoroquinolone resistance and dissemination

| Factor | Examples |
| --- | --- |
| Fluorquinolone usage | in humans and animals |
| Pharmacokinetic and pharmacodynamic factors | $AUC_{0-24}/MIC$<br>$C_{max}/MIC$<br>MPC and the mutant selection window |
| Clonal dissemination | infection control in hospitals<br>lack of clean water and poor sanitation<br>inadequate disease control programs<br>international transport of food<br>international travel of humans |

the United States increased by about 40% and was associated with a doubling in the rate of resistance to ciprofloxacin among Gram-negative bacilli isolated from hospital intensive care units [46]. In a retrospective study of fluoroquinolone use in 10 US teaching hospitals between 1991 and 2000, susceptibility to fluoroquinolones decreased significantly over the 10-year period, with particularly marked decreases in *P. aeruginosa* (25.1%), *Proteus mirabilis* (11.9%) and *E. coli* (6.8%) [73]. The increase in resistance was more than 50% in 5 of the 10 hospitals and there was a significant relationship between increasing levels of use and increasing levels of resistance ($p < 0.05$). In another study in 17 US hospitals, total fluoroquinolone use in the community was significantly associated with the percentage of *E. coli* isolates that were fluoroquinolone resistant ($r = 0.68$, $p = 0.003$) [74].

A similar relationship has been proposed between use and resistance for *S. pneumoniae*. In a case-control study in Hong Kong, multivariate analysis showed that presence of chronic obstructive pulmonary disease (OR 10.3), nosocomial origin of the bacteria (OR 16.2), residence in a nursing home (OR 7.4) and exposure to fluoroquinolones (OR 10.7) were independently associated with colonization or infection with levofloxacin-resistant pneumococci [75]. In a further study over various geographical regions in the United States, which used antimicrobial surveillance data, the levofloxacin MIC increased between 1997 and 2002, an increase that was significantly associated with levofloxacin usage across all regions ($p < 0.001$) [76].

The relationship between fluoroquinolone use in animal husbandry and resistance in non-typhoidal *Salmonella* serovars and *Campylobacter* has been the subject of considerable debate [77]. Fluoroquinolones, such as sarafloxacin and enrofloxacin, have been licensed for use in food animals (principally cattle, swine, poultry and fish), and companion animals. They are used for treatment, but also occasionally for growth promotion. Antimicrobials are, of necessity, often given on a group or flock-wide basis, rather than by administration to individual animals, and this may result in individual animals receiving sub-therapeutic doses. There is cross resistance between fluoroquinolones used specifically in animals and those used in human practice [78]. Furthermore, in some countries, fluoroquinolones used for humans are also used in animals. Most authorities now agree that animals are the principal source of quinolone-resistant isolates of *S. enterica* and *Campylobacter* spp. [79]. Epidemiological and laboratory data from a number of countries implicate fluoroquinolone use in poultry as a prime driver of resistance to quinolones among *C. jejuni* from humans [80], and its use in a variety of animals as a driver of resistance in non-Typhi *Salmonella* [37] and perhaps also *E. coli* [81].

Appropriate dosing regimens are critical for adequate therapy, but also for preventing the emergence of resistance. In recent years there has been a clearer understanding of the important pharmacokinetic and pharmacodynamic parameters. The ratio of the free drug area under the pharmacokinetic concentration-time curve and the MIC ($AUC_{0-24}$/MIC) and the ratio of the maximum drug concentration and the MIC ($C_{max}$/MIC) are both important determinants of bacterial eradication and resistance prevention for fluoroquinolones [82]. In one study of nosocomial lower respiratory tract infections the probabability of developing resistance during therapy increased significantly when antimicrobial exposure was at an $AUC_{0-24}$/MIC ratio of less than 100 [83]. A further useful parameter is the mutant protection concentration. This is a measure of the ability of bacteria to acquire resistance to quinolones by mutation [84]. When a large inoculum of bacteria ($10^{10}$) is plated on concentrations of a quinolone that are above its MIC, and the surviving bacteria are counted after 3 days of incubation, the lowest concentration at which no resistant mutants are obtained is called the MPC. The range of concentrations at which single-mutant selection may occur, the mutant selection window, lies between the MIC and the MPC. To minimize the selection of resistant mutants, it is suggested that the optimum quinolone regimen should have the narrowest mutant selection window and exceed the MPC for a significant proportion of the dosage interval. If the bacteria have decreased susceptibility to fluoroquinolones at the outset, the MPC will be higher making the acquisition of a further mutation and clinically significant resistance easier. MPC values for different strains of *Salmonella* with ciprofloxacin and enrofloxacin vary between 2 and 64 times the MIC [85]. Traditional drug dosages focus on killing susceptible cells, but run the risk of allowing the enrichment of drug-resistant mutants when the drug is in the mutant selection window. The implication of these pharmacokinetic/pharmacodynamic approaches is that doses required to cure the patient are lower than those required to prevent resistance. An increased risk of toxic side-effects, however, is the potential down-side of slowing the acquisition of resistance in a community by using higher doses.

Initial infection with a fluoroquinolone-resistant isolate is probably more common than resistance emerging during therapy. When a resistant strain has emerged, and provided its fitness is comparable with susceptible strains, dissemination becomes a critical part of the spread of resistance in an area [86, 87]. Once established in a community, a resistant strain of typhoid, for example, can rapidly spread from person to person or in the water supply [86]. The significant increase in post-treatment fecal carriage seen with fluoroquinolone treatment of nalidixic acid-resistant typhoid compared with nalidixic acid-susceptible strains, provides a selective advantage that encourages it to spread [15]. Linkage of fluoroquinolone resistance with resistance to other agents gives the strain a further advantage by allowing its selection by many antimicrobials. Local spread may be followed by international spread. The spread of non-Typhi *Salmonella* serovars illustrates the importance of the foreign travel and the international transport of food in the dissemination of resistant strains worldwide [32, 33]. Fluoroquinolone resistance in international clones of *S. pneumoniae* such as Spain[23F]-1 may also lead to widespread dissemination [55, 87].

## Conclusion

Decreased susceptibility and full resistance to fluoroquinolones has emerged or is emerging in many bacteria of considerable public health importance. This fall in susceptibility has implications for the management of individual patients and also has important public health outcomes both in hospitals and in the community. A variety of factors are driving this rise in resistance. Appropriate use of fluoroquinolones (and other antimicrobials) in humans and animals is urgently needed. The recent withdrawal of enrofloxacin use in poultry in the United States is a step in the right direction [88]. Care is required in the design of dosage regimens that cure patients and prevent resistance development. Adjustment of the breakpoints, to detect first-stage resistance mechanisms in bacteria such as *Salmonella* is long overdue, although will have important implications as alternative treatments are often limited. When resistant strains do emerge, well functioning hospital infection control and community disease control programs are critical to prevent their subsequent dissemination.

## References


1 Linder JA, Huang ES, Steinman MA, Gonzales R, Stafford RS: Fluoroquinolone prescribing in the United States: 1995 to 2002. Am J Med 2005;118:259–268.

2 Shankar PR, Upadhyay DK, Mishra P, Subish P, Dubey AK, Saha AC: Fluoroquinolone utilization among inpatients in a teaching hospital in Western Nepal. J Pakistan Med Assoc 2007;57:78–82.

3 Andriole VT: The Quinolones: past, present and future. Clin Infect Dis 2005;41(suppl 2):S113–S119.

4 Jacoby GA: Mechanisms of resistance to quinolones. Clin Infect Dis 2005;41:S120–S126.

5 Eliopoulos GM: Quinolone resistance mechanisms in pneumococci. Clin Infect Dis 2004;38(suppl 4): S350–S356.

6 Wang H, Dzink-Fox JL, Chen M, Levy SB: Genetic characterisation of highly fluoroquinolone-resistant *Escherichia coli* strains from China: role of *acrR* mutations. Antimicrob Agents Chemother 2001;45: 1515–1521.

7 Oethinger M, Kern W, Jellen-Ritter AS, McMurry LM, Levy SB: Ineffectiveness of topisomerase mutations in mediating clinically significant fluoroquinolone resistance in *Escherichia coli* in the absence of the AcrAB efflux pump. Antimicrob Agents Chemother 2000;44:10–13.

8 Robicsek A, Jacoby GA, Hooper DC: The world-wide emergence of plasmid-mediated quinolone resistance. Lancet Infect Dis 2006;6:629–640.

9 Robicsek A, Strahilevitz J, Jacoby GA, Macielag M, Abbanat D, Park CH, Bush K, Hooper DC: Fluor-quinolone-modifying enzyme: a new adaption of a common aminoglycoside acetyltransferase. Nat Med 2006;12:83–88.

10 Lindgren PK, Karlsson Å, Hughes D: Mutation rate and evolution of fluoroquinolone resistance in *Escherichia coli* isolates from patients with urinary tract infections. Antimicrob Agents Chemother 2003;47:3222–3232.

11 National Committee for Clinical Laboratory Standards: Performance standards for antimicrobial disk susceptibility tests; Approved Standard, ed 8. Document M2-A8, vol 20. Villanova, NCCLS, 2003.

12 British Society for Antimicrobial Chemotherapy: BSAC methods for antimicrobial susceptibility testing, version 6.1. 2007. Available at www.bsac.org.uk/_db/_documents/version_6.1.pdf (accessed September 3, 2009).

13 Aarestrup FM, Wiuff C, Mølbak K, Threlfall EJ: Is it time to change fluoroquinolone breakpoints for *Salmonella* spp? Antimicrob Agents Chemother 2003;47:827–829.

14 Crump JA, Barrett TJ, Nelson JT, Angulo FJ: Re-evaluating fluoroquinolone breakpoints for *Salmonella enterica* serotype Typhi and for non-Typhi Salmonellae. Clin Infect Dis 2003;37:75–81.

15 Parry CM: The treatment of multidrug resistant and nalidixic acid resistant typhoid fever in Vietnam. Trans Roy Soc Trop Med Hyg 2004;98:413–422.

16 Hakanen A, Kotilainen P, Jalava J, Siitonen A, Huovinen P: Detection of decreased fluoroquinolone susceptibility in Salmonellas and validation of nalidixic acid screening test. J Clin Microbiol 1999;37:3572–3577.

17 Cooke FJ, Day M, Wain J, Ward LR, Threlfall EJ: Cases of typhoid fever imported into England, Scotland and Wales (2000–2003). Trans Roy Soc Trop Med Hyg 2007;101:398–404.

18 Maskey AP, Day JN, Tuan PQ, Thwaites GE, Campbell JI, Zimmerman M, Farrar JJ, Basnyat B: *Salmonella enterica* serotype Paratyphi A and *S. enterica* serotype Typhi cause indistinguishable clinical syndromes in Kathmandu, Nepal. Clin Infect Dis 2006;42:1247–1253.

19 Renuka K, Kapil A, Kabra SK, Wig N, Das BK, Prasad VVSP, Chaudhry R, Seth P: Reduced susceptibility to ciprofloxacin and *gyrA* gene mutations in north Indian strains of *Salmonella enterica* serotype Typhi and serotype Paratyphi A. Microb Drug Resist 2004;10:146–153.

20 Walia M, Gaind R, Mehta R, Paul P, Aggarwal P, Kalaivani M: Current perspectives of enteric fever: a hospital based study from India. Ann Trop Paed 2005;25:161–174.

21 Rodrigues C, Mehta A, Joshi VR: *Salmonella Typhi* in the past decade: learning to live with resistance. Clin Infect Dis 2002;34:126.

22 Ahmed D, D'Costa LT, Alam K, Nair GB, Hossain MA: Multidrug-resistant *Salmonella enterica* serovar Typhi isolates with high-level resistance to ciprofloxacin in Dhaka, Bangladesh. Antimicrob Agents Chemother 2006;50:3516–3517.

23 Kariuki S, Revathi G, Muyodi J, Mwituria Jmunyalo A, Mirza S, Hart CA: Characterization of multidrug-resistant typhoid outbreaks in Kenya. J Clin Microbiol 2004;42:1477–1482.

24 Threlfall EJ, Fisher IST, Berghold C, Gerner-Smidt P, Tschäpe H, Comican M, Luzzi I, Schneider F, Wannet W, Machado J, Edwards G: Trends in antimicrobial resistance in *Salmonella enterica* serotypes Typhi and Paratyphi A isolated in Europe, 1999–2001. Int J Antimicrob Agents 2003;22:487.

25 Nair S, Unnikrishnan M, Turner K, Parija SC, Churcher C, Wain J, Harish BN: Molecular analysis of fluoroquinolone-resistant *Salmonella* Paratyphi A isolate, India. Emerg Infect Dis 2006;12:489–491.

26 Hasan R, Cooke FJ, Nair S, Harish BN, Wain J: Typhoid and paratyphoid fever. Lancet 2005;366: 1603–1604.

27 Renuka K, Sood S, Bas BK, Kapil A: High-level ciprofloxacin resistance in *Salmonella enterica* serotype Typhi in India. J Med Microbiol 2005;54:999–1000.

28 Saha SK, Darmstadt GL, Baqui AH, Crook DW, Islam MN, Islam M, Hossain M, Arifeen SE, Santosham M, Black RE: Molecular basis of resistance displayed by highly ciprofloxacin-resistant *Salmonella enterica* serovar Typhi in Bangladesh. J Clin Microbiol 2006;44:3811–3813.

29 Gaind R, Paglietti B, Murgia M, Dawar R, Uzzau S, Cappuccinelli P, Deb M, Aggarwal P, Rubino S: Molecular characterisation of ciprofloxacin-resistant *Salmonella enterica* serovar Typhi and Paratyphi A causing enteric fever in India. J Antimicrob Chemother 2006;58:1139–1144.

30 Stevenson JE, Gay K, Barrett TJ, Medalla F, Chiller TM, Angulo FJ: Increase in nalidixic acid resistance among non-Typhi *Salmonella enterica* isolates in the United States from 1996–2003. Antimicrob Agents and Chemother 2007;51:195–197.

31 Threlfall EJ, Fisher IST, Berghold C, et al: Antimicrobial drug resistance in isolates of *Salmonella enterica* from cases of salmonellosis in humans in Europe in 2000: results of international multi-centre surveillance. Eurosurveillance 2003;8:41–45.

32 Molbak K, Gerner-Smidt P, Wegener HC. Increasing quinolone resistance in *Salmonella enterica* serotype Enteritidis. Emerg Infect Dis 2002;8:514–515.

33 Hakanen A, Kotilainen P, Pitkänen S, Hillo S, Siitonen A, Houvinen P: Reductions in fluoroquinolone susceptibility among strains of *Salmonella enterica* isolated from Finnish patients. J Antimicrob Chemother 2006;57:569–572.

34 Soler P, González-Sanz R, Bleda MJ, Hernández G, Echeíta A, Usera MA: Antimicrobial resistance in non-typhoidal *Salmonella* from human sources, Spain, 2001–2203. J Antimicrob Chemother 2006; 58:310–314.

35 Choi SH, Woo JH, Lee JE, Park SJ, Choo EJ, Kwak YG, Kim MN, Choi MS, Lee NY, Lee BK, Kim NJ, Jeong JY, Ryu J, Kim YS: Increasing incidence of quinolone resistance in human non-typhoid *Salmonella enterica* isolates in Korea and mechanisms involved in quinolone resistance. J Antimicrob Chemother 2005;56:1111–1114.

36 Chiu CH, Wu TL, Su LH, et al: The emergence in Taiwan of fluoroquinolone resistance in *Salmonella enterica* serotype Choleraesuis. N Engl J Med 2002; 346:413–419.

37 Hsueh PR, Teng LJ, Tseng SP, Chang CF, Wan JH, Yan JJ, Lee CM, Chuang YC, Huang WK, Yang D, Shyr JM, Yu KW, Wang LS, Lu, JJ, Ko WC, Wu JJ, Chang FY, Yang YC, Lau YJ, Liu YC, Liu CY, Ho SW, Luh KT: Ciprofloxacin-resistant *Salmonella enterica* Typhimurium and Choleraesuis from pigs to humans, Taiwan. Emerg Infect Dis 2004;10:60–68.

38 Chiu, CH., Su LH, Chu C, Chia JH, Wu TL, Lin TY, Lee YS, Ou JT: Isolation of *Salmonella enterica* serotype Choleraesuis resistant to ceftriaxone and ciprofloxacin. Lancet 2004;363:1285–1286.

39 Chen S, Cui S, McDermott PF, Zhao S, White DG, Paulsen I, Meng J: Contribution of target gene mutations and efflux into decreased susceptibility of *Salmonella enterica* serovar Typhimurium to fluoroquinolones and other antimicrobials. Antimicrob Agents Chemother 2007;51:535–542.

40 Gay K, Robicsek A, Strahilevitz J, Park CH, Jacoby G, Barrett TJ, Medalla F, Chiller TM, Hooper DC: Plasmid mediated quinolone resistance in non-Typhi serotypes of *Salmonella enterica*. Clin Infect Dis 2006;43:297–304.

41 Hopkins KL, Wootton L, Day MR, Threlfall EJ: Plasmid-mediated mediated quinolone resistant determinant *qnrS1* found in *Salmonella enterica* strains in the UK. J Antimicrob Chemother 2007;59: 1071–1075.

42 Bachoual R, Ouabdesselam S, Mory F, Lascols C, Soussy CJ, Tankovic J: Single or double mutational alterations of gyrA associated with fluoroquinolone resistance in *Campylobacter jejuni* and *Campylobacter coli*. Microb Drug Resist 2001;7:257–261.

43 Gaunt PN, Piddock LJ: Ciprofloxacin resistant *Campylobacter* spp. in humans: an epidemiological and laboratory study. J Antimicrob Chemother 1996;37:747–757.

44 Centers for Disease Control and Prevention: National Antimicrobial Resistance Monitoring System: enteric bacteria. Atlanta, CDC, 2004. Accessed at www.cdc. gov/narms/annual/2004/NARMSAnnualReport2004. pdf (accessed September 3, 2009).

45 Gupta A, Nelson JM, Barrett TJ, Tauxe RV, Rossiter SP, Friedman CR, Joyce KW, Smith KE, Jones TF, Hawkins MA, Shiferaw B, Beebe JL, Vugia DJ, Rabatsky-Her T, Benson JA, Root TP, Angulo FJ: Antimicrobial resistance among *Campylobacter* strains, United States, 1997–2001. Emerg Infect Dis 2004;10:1102–1109.

46 Neuhauser MM, Weinstein RA, Rydman R, Danziger LH, Karam G, Quinn JP: Antibiotic resistance among Gram-negative bacilli in US intensive care units: implications for fluoroquinolone use. JAMA 2003;289:885–888.

47 Livermore DM, James D, Reacher M, Graham C: Trends in fluoroquinolone (ciprofloxacin) resistance in *Enterobacteriacae* from bacteraemias, England and Wales, 1990–1999. Emerg Infect Dis 2002; 5:473–478.

48 Paterson DL, Mulazimoglu L, Casellas JM, Ko W-C, Goossens H, von Gottberg A, Mohapatra S, Trenholme GM, Klugman KP, McCormack JG, Yu VL: Epidemiology of ciprofloxacin resistance and its relationship to extended-spectrum β-lactamase production in *Klebsiella* pneumoniae isolates causing bacteraemia. Clin Infect Dis 2000;30:473–478.

49 Lautenbach E, Strom BL, Bilker WB, Patel JB, Edelstein PH, Fishman NO. Epidemiological investigation of fluoroquinolone resistance in infections due to extended spectrum β-lactamase producing *Escherichia coli* and *Klebsiella pneumoniae*. Clin Infect Dis 2001;33:1288–1294.

50 Tapsall JW: Antibiotic resistance in *Neisseria gonorrhoeae*. Clin Infect Dis. 2005;41(suppl 4):S263–S268.

51 The WHO Western Pacific Surveillance Program: Surveillance of antibiotic resistance in *Neisseria gonorrhoeae* in the WHO Western Pacific Region, 2004. Commun Dis Intell 2006;30:129–132.

52 Centers for Disease Control and Prevention: Update to CDC's sexually transmitted diseases treatment guidelines, 2006: fluoroquinolones no longer recommended for treatment of gonococcal infections. MMWR 2007;56:332–336.

53 Martin IMC, Hoffmann S, Ison CA: European surveillance of sexually transmitted infections (ESSTI): the first combined antimicrobial susceptibility data for *Neisseria gonorrhoeae* in Western Europe. J Antimicrob Chemother 2006;58:587–593.

54   Adam HJ, Schurek KN, Nichol KA, Hoban CJ, Baudry TJ, Laing NM, Hoban DJ, Zhanel GG: Molecular characterisation of increasing fluoroquinolone resistance in *Streptococcus pneumoniae* isolates in Canada, 1997 to 2005. Antimicrob Agents Chemother 2007;51:198–207.

55   Ip M, Chaus SS, Chi CF, Cheuk ESC, Ma, H, Lai RWM, Chan PK: Longitudinally tracking fluoroquinolone resistance and its determinants in penicillin-susceptible and –nonsusceptible *Streptococcus pneumoniae* isolates in Hong Kong, 2000 to 2005. Antimicrob Agents and Chemother 2007;51:2192–2194.

56   Rupali P, Abraham OC, Jesudason MV, John TJ, Zachariah A, Sivaram S, Mathai D: Treatment failure in typhoid fever with ciprofloxacin susceptible *Salmonella enterica* serotype Typhi. Diagn Microbiol Infect Dis 2004;49:1–3.

57   Parry CM, Ho VA, Phuong LT, Bay PVB, Lanh MN, Tung LT, Tham TH, Wain J, Hien TT, Farrar JJ: Randomized controlled comparison of ofloxacin, azithromycin, and an ofloxacin-azithromycin combination for treatment of multidrug-resistant and nalidixic acid resistant typhoid fever. Antimicrob Agents Chemother 2007;51:819–825.

58   Mølbak K, Baggesen DL, Aarestrup FM, Ebbesen JM, Engberg J, Frydendahl K, Gerner-Smidt P, Petersen AM, Wegener HC: An outbreak of multidrug-resistant, quinolone resistant *Salmonella enterica* serotype Typhimurium DT104. N Engl J Med 1999;341:1420–1425.

59   Rahman M, Alam A, Nessa K, Nahar S, Dutta DK, Yasmin L, Monira S, Sultan Z, Khan A, Albert MJ: Treatment failure with the use of ciprofloxacin for gonorrhoeae correlates with the prevalence of fluoroquinolone-resistant Neisseria gonorrhoeae strains in Bangladesh. Clin Infect Dis 2001;32:884–889.

60   Aplasca De Los Reyes MR, Pato-Mesola V, Klausner JD, Manalastas R, Wi T, Tuazon CU, Dallbetta G, Whittington WL, Holmes KK: A randomized trial of ciprofloxacin versus cefixime for treatment of gonorrhoea after rapid emergence of gonococcal ciprofloxacin resistance in The Philippines. Clin Infect Dis 2001;32:1313–1318.

61   Davidson R, Cavalcanti R, Brunton JL, Bast DJ, de Azavedo JCS, Kibsey P, Flemming, Low DE: Resistance to levofloxacin and failure of treatment of pneumococcal pneumonia. N Engl J Med 2002;346:747–750.

62   Fuller JD, Low DE: A review of *Streptococcus pneumoniae* infection treatment failures associated with fluoroquinolone resistance. Clin Infect Dis 2005;41:118–121.

63   Mermin JH, Villar R, Carpenter J, Roberst L, Samaridden A, Gassanova L, Lomakina S, Bopp C, Hutwagner L, Mead P, Ross B, Mintz ED: A massive epidemic of multidrug-resistant typhoid fever in Tajikistan associated with consumption of municipal water. J Infect Dis 1999;179:1416–1422.

64   Olsen SJ, DeBess EE, McCivern TE, Marano N, Eby T, Maubais S, Balan VK, Zirnstein G, Cieslak PR, Angulo FJ: A nosocomial outbreak of fluoroquinolone-resistant *Salmonella* infection. N Engl J Med 2001;344:1572–1579.

65   Weiss K, Restieri C, Gauthier R, Laverdière M, McGreer A, Davidson RJ, Kilburn L, Bast DJ, de Azevado J, Low DE: A nosocomial outbreak of fluoroquinolone-resistant *Streptococcus pneumoniae*. Clin Infect Dis 2001;33:517–522.

66   Helms M, Vastrup P, Gerner-Smidt P, Mølbak K: Excess mortality associated with antimicrobial drug-resistant *Salmonella* Typhimurium. Emerg Infect Dis 2002;8:490–495.

67   Helms M, Simonsen J, Mølbak K: Quinolone resistance is associated with increased risk of invasive illness or death during infection with *Salmonella* serotype Typhimurium. J Infect Dis 2004;190:1652–1654.

68   Paterson DL: 'Collateral damage' from cephalosporin or quinolone antibiotic therapy. Clin Infect Dis 2004;38(suppl 4):S341–S345.

69   Pépin J, Saheb N, Coulombe MA, Alary ME, Corriveau MP, Authier S, LeBlanc M, Rivard G, Bettez M, Primeau V, Nguyen M, Jacob CE, Lanthier L: Emergence of fluoroquinolones as the predominant risk factor for *Clostridium difficile*-associated diarrhea: a cohort study during an epidemic in Quebec. Clin Infect Dis 2005;41:1254–1260.

70   LeBlanc L, Pépin J, Toulouse K, Ouellette MF, Coulombe MA, Corriveau MP, Alary ME: Fluoroquinolones and risk for methicillin-resistant *Staphylococcus aureus*, Canada. Emerg Infect Dis 2006;12:1398–1405.

71   Barza M, Travers K: Excess infections due to antimicrobial resistance: the 'attributable fraction'. Clin Infect Dis 2002;34(suppl 3):S126–S130.

72   Peña C, Albareda JM, Pallares R, Pujol M, Tubau F, Ariza J: Relationship between quinolone use and emergence of ciprofloxacin-resistant *Escherichia coli* in bloodstream infections. Antimicrob Agents Chemother 1995;39:520–524.

73   Zervos MJ, Hershberger E, Nicolau DP, Ritchie DJ, Blackner LK, Coyle EA, Donnelly AJ, Eckel SF, Eng RHK, Hilz A, Kuyumjian AG, Krebs W, McDaniel A, Hogan P, Lubowski TJ: Relationship between fluoroquinolone use and changes in susceptibility to fluoroquinolones of selected pathogens in 10 United States teaching hospitals, 1991–2000. Clin Infect Dis 2003;37:1643–1648.

74 MacDougall C, Powell JP, Johnson CK, Edmond MB, Polk RE: Hospital and community fluoroquinolone use and resistance in *Staphylococcus aureus* and *Escherichia coli* in 17 US hospitals. Clin Infect Dis 2005;41:435–440.

75 Ho PL, Tse WS, Tsang KWT, Ng TK, Cheng VCC, Chan RMT: Risk factors for acquisition of levofloxacin-resistant *Streptococcus pneumoniae*: a case-control study. Clin Infect Dis 2001;32:701–707.

76 Bhavnani SM, Hammel JP, Jones RN, Ambrose PG: Relationship between levofloxacin use and decreased susceptibility of *Streptococcus pneumoniae* in the United States. Diagn Microbiol Infect Dis 2005; 51:31–37.

77 Molbak K: Spread of resistant bacteria and resistance genes from animals to humans – The public health consequences. J Vet Med B 2004;51:364–369.

78 McDonald LC, Chen MT, Lauderdale TL, Ho M: The use of antibiotics critical to human medicine in food-producing animals in Taiwan. J Microbiol Immunol Infect 2001;34:97–102.

79 Food and Drug Administration: Risk assessment on the human health impact of fluoroquinolone resistant *Campylobacter* associated with the consumption of chicken. 2000 (revised 2001). www.fda.gov/Animal Veterinary/SafetyHealth/AntimicrobialResistance/ ucm083488.htm (accessed December 18, 2007).

80 Smith KE, Besser JM, Hedberg CW, Leano FT, Bender JB, Wicklund JH, Johnson BP, Moore KA, Osterholm MT: Quinolone-resistant *Campylobacter jejuni* infections in Minnesota, 1992–1998. N Engl J Med 1999;340:1525–1532.

81 Johnson JR, Kuskowski MA, Menard M, Gajewski A, Xercavins M, Garau J: Similarity between human and chicken *Escherichia coli* isolates in relation to ciprofloxacin resistance status. J Infect Dis 2006;194: 71–78.

82 Ambrose PG, Bhavnani SM, Rubino CM, Louie A, Gumbo T, Forrest A, Drusano GL: Pharmocokinetics-pharmacodynamics of antimicrobial therapy: it's not just for mice anymore. Clin Infect Dis 2007;44: 79–86.

83 Thomas JK, Forrest A, Bhavnani SM, Hyatt JM, Cheng A, Ballow CH, Schentag JJ: Pharmacodynamic evaluation of factors associated with the development of bacterial resistance in acutely ill patients during therapy. Antimicrob Agents Chemother 1998;42:521–527.

84 Drlica K, Zhao X: Mutant selection window hypothesis updated. Clin Infect Dis 2007;44:681–688.

85 Randall LP, Cooles SW, Piddock LJV, Woodward MJ: Mutant protection concentrations of ciprofloxacin and enrofloxacin for *Salmonella enterica*. J Antimicrob Chemother 2004;54:688–691.

86 Davis MA, Hancock DD, Besser TE: Multiresistant clones of *Salmonella enterica*: the importance of dissemination. J Lab Clin Med 2002;140:135–141.

87 Klugman K: The role of clonality in the global spread of fluoroquinolone-resistant bacteria. Clin Infect Dis 2003;36:783–785.

88 Nelson JM, Chiller TM, Powers JH, Angulo FJ: Fluoroquinolone-resistant *Campylobacter* species and the withdrawal of fluoroquinolones from use in poultry: a public heath success story. Clin Infect Dis 2007;44:977–980.

Christopher M. Parry
School of Infection and Host Defence
Faculty of Medicine, University of Liverpool
Duncan Building, Daulby Street, Liverpool L6 3GA (UK)
Tel. +44 151 706 4381, Fax +44 151 706 5805, E-Mail cmparry@liverpool.ac.uk

Weber JT (ed): Antimicrobial Resistance – Beyond the Breakpoint.
Issues Infect Dis. Basel, Karger, 2010, vol 6, pp 51–69

# Antibiotic Resistance and Community-Acquired Pneumonia during an Influenza Pandemic

Matthew R. Moore · Cynthia G. Whitney

Respiratory Diseases Branch, National Center for Immunization and Respiratory Diseases, Centers for Disease
Control and Prevention, Atlanta, Ga., USA

**Abstract**
The threat of an influenza pandemic in 2009 stimulated intense interest in pandemic preparedness,
including mobilization of local, state, federal and international resources. There were also discussions on non-pharmacologic approaches to containment and implementation of programs to stockpile neuraminidase inhibitors and vaccines against potential strains of pandemic influenza. All of
these activities are important components of preparedness in the United States. However, literature
published after each of the 20th century influenza pandemics shows that bacterial pneumonia following influenza infection was a major cause of morbidity and mortality. Some key differences
between those pandemics and the next one include characteristics of the individual pandemic
strains, the availability of antiviral agents, the availability of antibiotics and the prevalence of associated antimicrobial resistance among common bacterial etiologies of community-acquired pneumonia, and the availability of a protein-conjugate vaccine for *Haemophilus influenzae* type B disease and
2 vaccines that target *Streptococcus pneumoniae*. A key challenge posed by the next pandemic is
how best to use prevention strategies and antibiotics to minimize morbidity and mortality from secondary bacterial pneumonia.                    Copyright © 2010 S. Karger AG, Basel

## Epidemiology of Bacterial Community-Acquired Pneumonia During Inter-Pandemic Periods in the United States

The incidence of pneumonia follows a 'U'-shaped age distribution, occurring most
commonly in the very young and the very old. Most hospitalizations and deaths occur
among the elderly, who are more likely to have underlying illnesses that increase their
risk for severe infection [1]. The prevalences of specific etiologies of pneumonia also
vary somewhat with age [2]. Although pneumococcus is a common bacterial pathogen in all age groups, viruses such as respiratory syncytial virus are more common in
young children while *Mycoplasma pneumoniae* predominates in school-aged children
[3]. *Legionella*, the causative agent of Legionnaires' disease, tends to cause community-

acquired pneumonia (CAP) in the elderly and those with underlying immunosuppressive illnesses. Finally, *Staphylococcus aureus* and group A *Streptococcus* have long been recognized as important causes of CAP following influenza infection. Of the bacterial etiologies of CAP, *Streptococcus pneumoniae* and *Staphylococcus aureus* are the most common causes of secondary bacterial pneumonia among patients with influenza, and both frequently demonstrate resistance to antibiotics used for empiric treatment of CAP. Pneumonia in general and *S. pneumoniae* in particular share similar seasonal patterns with influenza [4–6]. In addition, *S. pneumoniae* and *S. aureus* are common colonizers of the upper respiratory tract [7, 8]. The remainder of this chapter will focus on these 2 organisms.

*Clinical Significance of Antimicrobial Resistance: S. pneumoniae*

Unequivocal evidence of bacteriologic or clinical failure as a direct result of antibiotic resistance is difficult to document for bacterial infections, including pneumococcal pneumonia [9]. For penicillins, it is difficult to demonstrate a clear relationship between resistance in the pneumococcus and clinical failure, perhaps because the susceptibility breakpoints were initially established on the basis of achievable levels of penicillin in the cerebrospinal fluid whereas most pneumococcal infections occur in the lung or the bloodstream. Two studies from Asia suggest that penicillin non-susceptibility is common, with 40–60% of pneumococcal strains classified as intermediate or fully resistant; however, reduced susceptibility could not be related to a worse clinical outcome [10, 11]. A recent international study failed to find a relationship between discordant therapy for pneumococcal pneumonia and mortality and, therefore, concluded that the use of penicillin therapy against penicillin non-susceptible strains does not increase the risk of mortality [12]. Pharmacokinetic data suggest that penicillin dosing may achieve levels in the blood higher than the minimum inhibitory concentrations (MICs) of most penicillin-resistant organisms [13]. Because of these studies and others [14–16], the susceptibility breakpoints for intravenous penicillin and non-meningitis cases of pneumococcal infection were recently increased. As a result, a higher proportion of pneumococcal pneumonia cases are now likely to be under the breakpoint, thus amenable to treatment with penicillin [17].

Cephalosporins are frequently used for empiric treatment of CAP and are often effective against penicillin-resistant strains of *S. pneumoniae*. However, treatment failures have been documented for first (cefazolin) [18], second (cefuroxime) [12, 19, 20], and third (ceftazidime) [21] generation cephalosporins. Cefotaxime and ceftriaxone, both third-generation agents, are recommended for empiric pneumonia therapy because the prevalence of resistance to these antibiotics is low and because there is little evidence that treatment of resistant strains with these antibiotics leads to poorer outcome [22–24].

Data suggesting a relationship between fluoroquinolone-resistant pneumococci and treatment failure appear to be mounting but are still limited to anecdotal episodes

[25–27]. A recent literature review identified 20 failures of ciprofloxacin and levoflox-acin therapy for respiratory infections caused by fluoroquinolone-resistant *S. pneumoniae* [28]. What distinguishes fluoroquinolones from other drug classes is that, in the United States and most other countries, fluoroquinolones are used rarely in children, the reservoir of pneumococcal colonization.

The class of drugs with the largest body of evidence suggesting that resistance leads to treatment failure is the macrolide class, including erythromycin and the new azolides, azithromycin and clarithromycin [29]. Klugman [27] recently highlighted that macrolide resistance among pneumococci appears to be increasing in prevalence, the MICs of existing macrolide resistant strains are increasing, and the MIC is a good predictor of treatment failure. A report from 5 years of surveillance in Toronto identi-fied 1,696 episodes of pneumococcal bacteremia, nearly two thirds of which presented as pneumonia. Of these, 3.5% were failures of outpatient macrolide or azolide therapy, and two thirds of the failures were caused by macrolide-resistant strains [30].


*Clinical Significance of Antimicrobial Resistance: S. aureus*


Some of the best evidence linking antimicrobial resistance among *S. aureus* to clini-cal treatment failure comes from studies of *S. aureus* infective endocarditis [31–34]. Methicillin-resistant *S. aureus* (MRSA) has emerged as a community pathogen in recent years and co-infections with influenza and *S. aureus* have been described [35]. However, determining the clinical significance of antimicrobial-resistant *S. aureus* – especially MRSA – causing pneumonia has been more challenging. Some descriptions of MRSA pneumonia among previously healthy individuals have been especially dra-matic, possibly due to the presence of Panton-Valentine leukocidin [36–42], a toxin thought to enhance the pathogenicity of strains expressing it or other virulence fac-tors such as staphylococcal protein A (Spa) [43]. Because of the rapidity with which these community-associated MRSA strains cause pneumonia and death, it may not be possible to determine whether methicillin resistance, independent of other factors, predicts treatment failure. Data comparing vancomycin to linezolid for the treatment of healthcare-associated *S. aureus* pneumonia has generated some debate as to which agent leads to the best clinical outcome [44].


## Biological Mechanisms for Interactions Between Influenza and Bacterial CAP

Influenza viruses promote bacterial infection at the cellular level in several ways. Experiments in the 1950s were the first to suggest that influenza virus may impair the ability of respiratory epithelium to clear bacteria [45]. More recent studies show that defects in phagocytic function [46, 47] during influenza infection permit increased bacterial replication and that the cytokine response to influenza leads to improved bacterial adherence and invasion with in vitro and animal models [48, 49]. Extensive studies by McCullers and colleagues have shown that the neuraminidase enzyme of influenza primes the lung for pneumococcal infection by increasing adherence of pneumococci to lung cells [48] and inhibition of the neuraminidase enzyme with neuraminidase inhibitors can reverse this effect in mice [50].

**Epidemiologic Evidence That Influenza Increases the Risk of Bacterial CAP**

*Inter-Pandemic Influenza*

Several types of evidence support an epidemiologic relationship between influenza infection and subsequent bacterial CAP. First, an ecologic relationship between influenza and CAP has been recognized for many years, with hospitalizations and deaths related to both diseases peaking simultaneously [51]. More direct evidence at the individual patient level was provided by a retrospective case-control study conducted in the context of an outbreak of severe pneumococcal disease among children. In that study, the investigators demonstrated a 12-fold increased risk of an influenza-like illness in the 7–28 days before hospitalization for pneumococcal pneumonia and a nearly 4-fold increased risk of a positive influenza A convalescent serology among patients with pneumococcal disease [52]. A more novel approach to the question of causality was taken in the context of a randomized, double-blind, placebo-controlled clinical trial of a protein-polysaccharide conjugate pneumococcal vaccine in South Africa. Children who had received pneumococcal vaccine experienced a risk of hospitalization for laboratory-confirmed influenza infection that was 45% lower than children who had received placebo, suggesting that the vaccine was directly preventing pneumococcal pneumonia as a complication of influenza infection [53]. Because influenza vaccine was not available during this trial, it is unknown whether both vaccines in combination would have further reduced influenza-associated hospitalizations.

With respect to CAP caused by *S. aureus*, Hageman recently reported 17 cases of culture-confirmed community-acquired *S. aureus* pneumonia among persons with either an influenza-like illness (i.e. fever plus sore throat or cough) or laboratory-confirmed influenza infection before onset of pneumonia symptoms [35]. Of the 13 cases from whom *S. aureus* isolates were available, 11 were methicillin resistant and 10 of these were identified as the USA300 strain, a pulsed-field gel electrophoresis type associated with severe necrotizing pneumonia [54].

*Pandemic Influenza*

Evidence supporting the relationship between influenza and bacterial CAP during previous pandemics far outweighs the evidence available from studies conducted during inter-pandemic periods [55]. Of the 3 influenza pandemics in the 20th century, 1 occurred in the pre-antibiotic era and all 3 occurred in the era before effective influenza and pneumococcal vaccines and influenza antiviral medications were available.

*1918–1919 Influenza Pandemic*

The 1918–1919 pandemic caused more illness and death than the other two 20th century pandemics combined. Approximately 500 million persons, one third of the world's population, were infected and 50–100 million persons died [56, 57]. A key determinant of the severity of that pandemic was the influenza virus itself, the virulence of which likely led to severe lung inflammation [58, 59].

In addition to the virulence of the influenza virus, bacterial pneumonia also likely played an important role in the elevated mortality observed in 1918–1919. During those years, the US Public Health Service conducted house-to-house surveys in 11 localities throughout the country (New London, Conn.; Baltimore and several combined communities, Md.; Spartanburg, S.C.; Augusta and Macon, Ga.; Louisville, Ky.; Little Rock, Ariz.; Des Moines, Iowa; San Antonio, Tex.; San Francisco, Calif.) [60]. While the population sampled was small – just over 130,000 persons total – the survey was very detailed and highlights key relationships between influenza and pneumonia not evident from other reports. The overall influenza attack rate varied widely, from 15% in Louisville to 54% in San Antonio with an average of 28% of persons reporting an influenza-like illness. Most of the geographic differences were attributed to different age distributions in each area, as age-specific influenza attack rates were quite similar across sites. Regardless of locality, incidence of influenza was not directly related to overall mortality. Instead, pneumonia incidence determined case-fatality rates which, in turn, determined overall mortality. In short, pneumonia as a complication of influenza was a key determinant of mortality.

Attack rates of secondary bacterial pneumonia during the 1918 pandemic ranged from 7.1% to 20%, depending on the phase of the pandemic and on the population studied [61]. For example, of the 63,374 soldiers at Fort Riley in Kansas, 15,170 (24%) developed influenza between September 15 and November 1. Of these, 2,624 (17%) developed pneumonia, of whom 941 (36%) died, for an overall death rate of 1.5% [62]. In Baltimore, 268 civilians with influenza were admitted to Johns Hopkins Hospital between September 24 and October 20, 1918. Of these, 41 (15.3%) developed pneumonia, among whom 13 (32%) died [63].

While diagnostic techniques used today were not available in 1918, published literature from that period includes descriptions of pre- and post-mortem examinations of clinical material that provide some insights into the common bacterial etiologies of CAP (table 1). The pneumococcus was clearly the most common bacterial etiology of pneumonia, appearing in roughly 40–70% of pre-mortem sterile-site specimens (e.g. blood, lung punctures) and 30–75% of post-mortem specimens (e.g. heart blood and lung tissue). Group A streptococci were also recovered from

**Table 1.** Percentages of CAP cases by etiologic agent during influenza pandemics, 1918–1968

| | Etiology | | | | Ref. |
|---|---|---|---|---|---|
| | *S. pneumoniae* | *H. influenzae* | Group A streptococci | *S. aureus* | |
| *Pre-mortem* | | | | | |
| Invasive | | | | | |
| Blood | 100 (45/45) | | | | [61, 122] |
| | 44 (23/52)[a] | | | | [123] |
| | 12 (6/50) | | | 0 (0/50) | [70] |
| Lung puncture | 73 (11/15) | | 19.8 (3/15) | | [124] |
| Non-invasive | | | | | |
| Sputum | 48 (52/108)[b] | 11 (12/108)[b] | | 19 (21/108)[b] | [69] |
| | 26 (191/740) | | 17 (126/740) | | [61, 125] |
| | 41 (65/158) | 38 (58/158) | 29 (46/158) | | [61, 126] |
| | 70 (70/100) | 4 (4/100) | | | [124] |
| | 27 (3/11) | 9 (1/11) | | | [127] |
| | 63 (24/38) | 16 (6/38) | | 16 (6/38) | [66] |
| | 43 (23/54) | | | 9 (5/54) | [70] |
| *Post-mortem* | | | | | |
| Lung tissue | 44 (4/9) | | | | [61, 128] |
| | 28 (77/280) | | 27 (76/280) | | [61, 125] |
| | 45 (9/20) | | | 20 (2/10) | [61, 126] |
| | | 8.8 (3/34) | | | [124] |
| | | | | 48 (153/312) | [61, 65] |
| | | | | 38 (12/32) | [68] |
| Pleural cavities | 67 (6/9) | | | | [61, 128] |
| Heart blood | 65 (52/82) | 2.5 (2/80) | 7.5 (6/82) | 1.3 (1/82) | [61, 129] |

| | Etiology | | | | Ref. |
|---|---|---|---|---|---|
| | *S. pneumoniae* | *H. influenzae* | Group A streptococci | *S. aureus* | |
| | 33 (3/9) | | | | [61, 128] |
| | 28 (77/280) | | 22 (62/280) | | [61, 125] |
| 'Necropsies' | | 43 (16/37) | | | [61, 129] |
| *Results not distinguished* | | | | | |
| Sputum and necropsy material | 9 (12/140) | 4 (5/140) | 1 (2/140) | 27 (38/140) | [67] |

Data are percentages of secondary bacterial pneumonia cases caused by each etiology. Numbers in parentheses are isolates/patients with specimens for culture.

[a] Isolates only identified as 'streptococci'.

[b] Report does not indicate what proportion came from each specimen source.

pre-mortem expectorated sputum specimens, although less commonly than pneumococci. *H. influenzae* ('Pfeiffer's Bacillus') was common enough in the 1918 and previous epidemics to suggest that it might have been the actual cause of influenza, a notion eventually dispelled with the isolation of influenza virus in 1933 [64].

The identification of *S. aureus* from autopsy specimens during the 1918–1919 pandemic suggests that it may have been associated with higher case fatality rates than other bacteria. In the autumn of 1918, 8,100 soldiers at Camp Jackson (S.C.) were admitted to hospital with influenza. Of these, 1,409 developed secondary bacterial pneumonia and 7–12% of these cases (depending on the regiment) were diagnosed as *S. aureus* pneumonia. While the case fatality rate of all-cause pneumonia at Camp Jackson was 27% (385/1409), *S. aureus* accounted for a disproportionate number of deaths. Of 312 post-mortem lung cultures obtained from soldiers 153 (49%), yielded growth of *S. aureus* either in pure culture or in combination with other bacteria, most commonly pneumococcus. In other words, pneumococcus was the most common cause of secondary bacterial pneumonia but *S. aureus* had a higher case fatality rate [65].

*1957–1958 Influenza Pandemic*

If the 1918–1919 pandemic demonstrated the natural history of bacterial pneumonia as a complication of influenza, the 1957–1958 (Asian) pandemic provided the first insight into the epidemiology of secondary bacterial pneumonia during the antibiotic era. One of the most detailed reports comes from New Haven Hospital in Connecticut where, in the autumn of 1957, 91 patients were admitted with radiographically or autopsy-confirmed pneumonia, a 6-fold increase in pneumonia admissions compared to the same period in 1956 [66]. The clinical histories of these patients confirmed the 1918 epidemiology in that many patients described the onset of influenza-like symptoms approximately 1 week before presenting to hospital for admission. Since the 1918–1919 pandemic, it has been well established that pregnant women are at increased risk of influenza-related complications. In 1957, however, this association manifested as increased risk of secondary bacterial pneumonia among pregnant women. Among males admitted with secondary bacterial pneumonia, more than half were aged 50 or older, emphasizing the role of co-morbidities in this population [67]. Among females, however, almost two thirds were between the ages of 16 and 40 and almost half of these were in their third trimester of pregnancy [66–68].

Because of the availability of antibiotics in 1957, most patients with bacterial pneumonia diagnosed by sputum smear and culture received antibiotics [68]. Penicillin was used to treat pneumococcal infections, streptomycin and chloramphenicol was used for *H. influenzae,* and all 3 drugs were used to treat *S. aureus* pneumonia. Only 11 (12%) patients with bacterial pneumonia in the New Haven sample died, a reduction in case-fatality of nearly two thirds compared to 1918. However, 7 of these 11 fatal cases had no underlying illnesses and in 4 fatal cases where a bacterial etiology was identified, 3 were caused by *S. aureus.* It is highly likely that differences in the influenza virus itself contributed to the lower mortality in 1957 compared to 1918. However, antibiotics also clearly benefited patients with pneumococcal pneumonia [66].

The 1957 pandemic also provided some insight into the relationship between time of hospitalization and the susceptibility of strains of *S. aureus.* Among 20 strains of *S. aureus* recovered from patients with pneumonia, 9 were recovered from patients upon admission and all of these were susceptible to penicillin, chloramphenicol, and streptomycin. Of the remaining 11 strains, which were recovered on average 1 week after admission, all were resistant to those same agents [67]. These data suggest that at least some, and up to half, of influenza-associated *S. aureus* pneumonia cases may be acquired in hospital.

Finally, the 1957 pandemic demonstrated how outpatient antibacterial therapy can impact the epidemiology of hospitalized CAP. In one report from Sheffield (UK) most patients with CAP received antibiotics before admission. Among the 140 patients hospitalized with CAP, an organism was recovered from sputum or at autopsy from 74 (53%). Unlike the pre-antibiotic era where pneumococci would have been recovered from roughly 50% of patients with a known etiology, pneumococcus was recovered from only 12 (9%) of patients. Instead, *S. aureus* was recovered from 27% of cases and Gram-negative organisms from another 12% [67]. Whether the high rate of recovery of *S. aureus* is related to the bias inherent in autopsy studies (i.e. inclusion of only cases resulting in death) is unclear; however, these data do suggest that outpatient antibiotic therapy can reduce the proportion of hospitalized secondary bacterial pneumonia cases with pneumococcus identified as an etiology.

*1968–1969 Influenza Pandemic*
Available literature from the 1968–1969 pandemic differs from the other 2 pandemics in that fewer reports in 1968–1969 relied on autopsy studies. It is unknown whether this observation is a result of decreased virulence of the 1968 influenza virus with substantially fewer influenza-related deaths overall compared to prior pandemics, fewer deaths from secondary bacterial pneumonia, a smaller proportion of those fatalities having autopsies performed, or some combination of these.

In January 1969, a large increase in the number of patients presenting to a hospital in Atlanta (Ga.) with acute respiratory infections prompted the adoption of a policy to admit all patients with clinical or radiographic evidence of pneumonia. Schwarzmann et al. [69] reviewed all 108 cases and found that pneumococcus was the most common etiology. This study also clarified the relationship between influenza and *S. aureus* by showing that the number of cases of *S. aureus* pneumonia increased, in relative terms, more than any other organism, from 6% of cases during the previous influenza season to 19% during the pandemic. In contrast, 61% of CAP cases were caused by pneumococcus during the previous influenza season compared to 48% during the pandemic [69]. In other words, pneumococcus was still the most common cause of secondary bacterial pneumonia during the pandemic but *S. aureus* demonstrated the largest increase in prevalence compared to the previous influenza season. Finally, 70% of *S. aureus* isolates were resistant to penicillin – a change from 1957 – while 100% were susceptible to oxacillin and cephalothin.

Between December 1968 and January 1969, 106 patients with clinical evidence of pneumonia were admitted to the City of Memphis (Tennessee) Hospitals, a system primarily for the indigent population of Memphis [70]. All but 2 of these patients also had radiographic evidence of pneumonia. Seventy-nine (75%) of all CAP patients had evidence of current or recent influenza infection, either by serology or viral isolation. Bisno et al. [70] established criteria for assigning etiologic diagnoses that were more stringent than those used in previous studies of hospitalized patients. These were: that all cases required serologic or culture evidence of influenza infection; none was permitted to have any history of antibiotic administration before admission, and all had bacterial cultures obtained before receiving antibacterial therapy in hospital. Of 54 patients meeting these criteria for influenza-associated CAP, 23 (43%) had pneumococcus isolated in pure culture from sputum and 5 (9%) had *S. aureus* isolated, most in mixed culture. Fifty of these same patients had blood cultures collected before antibiotic administration and 6 (12%) yielded pneumococci while none revealed *S. aureus*. Of note, Bisno et al. categorized their cases using Louria's classification. They were able to identify clearly all pulmonary syndromes with the exception of primary influenza pneumonia. As a potential explanation for the disagreement with Louria's study [71], Bisno noted that patients with rheumatic heart disease in Memphis in

1967 received monthly prophylaxis with benzathine penicillin, a measure which might have reduced their risk for secondary pneumococcal pneumonia.

*Etiologic Information from Influenza Pandemics: Interpretation and Summary*

Data published in the wake of all three 20th century pandemics suffer from a key limitation, namely, the inability to draw clear conclusions from results of imperfect diagnostic tests. Upper respiratory specimens are frequently colonized with either *S. pneumoniae* or *S. aureus*, leading potentially to the incorrect assignment of one etiology when the true etiology is something else. Conversely, reliance on blood cultures, which yield an organism in less than 20% of patients with CAP [72], may lead to an underestimate of the proportion of cases attributable to pneumococcus or *S. aureus*, especially in situations where patients have received antibiotics before blood cultures were obtained. Nevertheless, published studies describing the etiologies of secondary bacterial pneumonia during influenza pandemics are, on balance, consistent with each other and with other studies conducted during inter-pandemic years. These studies can be summarized as follows:

- Pneumococcus is the most common cause of secondary bacterial pneumonia during influenza pandemics.
- Relative to inter-pandemic years, *S. aureus* demonstrates the largest increase in prevalence of any one etiology during pandemics.
- *S. aureus* predominates in autopsy-based studies, suggesting that it might have a higher case fatality rate.
- Up to one half of secondary pneumonia cases caused by *S. aureus* during influenza pandemics may be acquired in hospital.

## Relationship Between Past and Future Pandemics

Given what we know about previous pandemics, a key challenge is to ensure that all patients with secondary bacterial pneumonia are treated appropriately with antibiotics while minimizing the inevitable consequences of promoting antibiotic resistance. By comparing previous pandemics to what might be expected from the next one, it might be possible to identify those questions which, if answered, could aid in preventing cases of secondary bacterial pneumonia, including those resistant to antibiotics.

*Similarities among Cases of Secondary Bacterial Pneumonia*

Similar to the 1968 pandemic, when antibiotics were widely available, we can expect that most patients with any evidence of CAP during a pandemic will be treated with antibiotics. We can also expect that there will be shortages of vaccines, antiviral and antibacterial agents, diagnostic test reagents and hospital beds [73, 74]. Anticipating these shortages as much as possible, preventing them and providing guidance on how to best manage patients during shortages are all critical steps for pandemic planning.

We should also expect that it will continue to be challenging to differentiate between primary viral, primary bacterial, and viral and bacterial co-infections as etiologies of pneumonia, a differentiation that is critical for deciding when antibiotics are indicated [75, 76]. However, recent advances in diagnostic techniques hold some promise that this important differentiation will become more feasible [77, 78]. Whether these techniques improve the ability to differentiate viral from bacterial etiologies in daily clinical practice and whether they can be implemented in community settings remains to be seen.

*Differences Between Previous and Future Pandemics*

One of the most important differences between the three 20th century pandemics and those of today and in the future is the availability of primary prevention strategies for influenza. Although supplies will likely be limited, antivirals [79–81] and influenza vaccines [82, 83] could prevent cases of pandemic influenza infection which would otherwise be complicated by secondary bacterial pneumonia.

Concomitant with the increasing age of the population, the prevalence of underlying illnesses that increase the risk of influenza and pneumonia has increased over the past century [51, 84, 85]. Little is known about the risk of influenza among persons living with HIV or AIDS [86–88]. However, pneumonia, including pneumococcal pneumonia, is clearly a major cause of morbidity and mortality in that population [89, 90]. Asthma, which has recently been shown to be a risk factor for invasive pneumococcal disease [91], has also increased in prevalence in recent years [92]. Conversely, the prevalence of smoking which has long been associated with pneumonia, and pneumococcal disease, has started to decline [93].

The introduction of protein-conjugate vaccine for *Haemophilus influenzae* B in the 1990s led to important reductions in this invasive disease [94]. During that same decade, the prevalence of antimicrobial-resistant *S. pneumoniae* in the United States increased dramatically [95]. This increase reversed following the introduction of pneumococcal conjugate vaccine into the routine infant immunization schedule. Whether this trend will continue or reverse yet again remains to be seen [96]. Perhaps the most novel aspect of a pandemic now or in the future will be the role of community-associated MRSA. As mentioned previously, the increase in prevalence of methicillin resistance among *S. aureus* isolates has become an important concern among clinicians, both because of the rate of increase in prevalence and because of the dramatic clinical presentations [36–38, 42, 54, 73].

The relationship between diagnostic testing and antibiotic use is also somewhat different today compared to during previous pandemics. Non-culture-based methods such as urine antigen tests or nucleic acid-based tests were not available during previous pandemics but both are now recommended for use in CAP, at least among adults [97]. At the same time clinical practices have moved away from culture-based tests [98], perhaps because empiric therapies currently available are broad spectrum, safe and highly effective [99].

Despite all that is known from previous pandemics, there is much that cannot be predicted. What proportion of the population will develop pandemic influenza infection? What proportion of those will develop secondary bacterial pneumonia? What proportion of cases of pneumonia will have an etiology identified and what proportion of those will be antimicrobial resistant? Previous pandemics can provide some clues to the answers [55, 60] but those clues need to be interpreted with cautious skepticism.

**Strategies for Reducing Secondary Pneumonia Caused by Resistant Bacteria during a Pandemic**

Several strategies might reduce the burden of antimicrobial resistant secondary bacterial pneumonia during a pandemic. Strategies aimed at reducing the incidence of influenza infection could markedly reduce episodes of secondary bacterial pneumonia. These include use of antiviral agents, influenza vaccines and social distancing measures. There is also some evidence to support strategies that could limit unnecessary antibiotic use even when prior influenza infection is suspected. Previous pandemics suggest that patients who appear relatively well and do not have significant findings on chest radiographs will not benefit from antibiotics [71]. Although clinicians over-prescribe antibiotics for patients with clinical signs of pneumonia [100], results of radiographs, when provided to clinicians, can reduce antibiotic use among patients suspected of having pneumonia from 43 to 17% [101].

When radiographic evidence of pneumonia is present, clinicians can reduce unnecessary prescribing through efforts to identify the bacterial etiology. Numerous studies have shown that clinicians cannot distinguish between specific etiologies of CAP based on clinical criteria alone [72, 102]. However, identifying that the etiology is a virus alone instead of a bacterium or a co-infection with both – without identifying the specific organism – could allow clinicians to reassure their patients that antibiotics are not indicated. Use of surrogate markers of inflammation, such as procalcitonin and C-reactive protein, holds some promise for targeting antimicrobials for patients most likely to have bacterial infections [103, 104].

When antibiotics are prescribed for documented episodes of pneumonia, prescribing the narrowest possible antimicrobial for the most likely infection may help to prevent the development of resistance. In recent years a debate has developed over whether dual therapy with a cephalosporin and a macrolide might reduce mortality among patients hospitalized with pneumococcal pneumonia [105, 106]. Whether this benefit exists is unclear [15] and, if so, whether it is related to immunomodulating effects of macrolide drugs or to the effects of macrolides on co-infecting atypical organisms. In either case, use of extended spectrum macrolides has been associated with the promotion of resistance [107, 108]; therefore, determining whether patients with secondary bacterial pneumonia should also receive dual therapy will be important. Finally, there may be clinical situations in which short course therapy will be appropriate [109] and these regimens could forestall the development of resistance.

The role of antibacterial vaccines for the prevention of secondary bacterial pneumonia is also a critical concern. While there are no vaccines currently licensed for prevention of *S. aureus* infections, pneumococcal vaccines were studied as early as 1918 [110] and continued among South African gold miners where a pneumococcal vaccine targeting 14 serotypes was shown to prevent pneumococcal pneumonia [111]. Since that trial, however, there has been some debate about whether pneumococcal polysaccharide vaccines are effective at preventing pneumococcal pneumonia without bacteremia, with most studies being unable to document benefit [112]. Regardless, pneumococcal polysaccharide vaccine has been shown to have 50–80% effectiveness against invasive pneumococcal disease caused by serotypes included in the vaccine, depending on the study and the population [113–115]. Again, given the burden of secondary pneumococcal pneumonia during the next pandemic, efforts to improve coverage with the currently recommended 23-valent pneumococcal polysaccharide vaccine could have substantial public health benefits [116, 117].

The availability of the 7-valent pneumococcal conjugate vaccine (PCV7) holds great promise from several different perspectives. First, PCV7 has been shown to reduce dramatically rates of invasive pneumococcal disease, including antibiotic resistant infections, among children and adults [96, 118]. Fewer cases of pneumococcal disease means fewer antibiotic prescriptions [119]. Finally, PCV7 has been shown to reduce rates of antibiotic-resistant invasive pneumococcal disease, not only in the children for whom the vaccine is recommended but also among adults who benefit from the herd immunity conferred by the vaccine [96]. An application for a 13-valent conjugate vaccine is being reviewed by regulatory authorities in the United States and Europe.

Given the role that hospital-acquired resistant *S. aureus* infections may have played in previous pandemics, basic infection control procedures are critical for preventing healthcare-associated *S. aureus* infections during the next pandemic. These procedures include staff education, infection and microbiologic surveillance, preventing transmission of bacterial etiologies of pneumonia, and modifying the host's risk for infection [120, 121].

**Table 2.** Interventions for the prevention of community-acquired, antibiotic-resistant secondary bacterial pneumonia during an influenza pandemic

---

- Where available, administer influenza vaccines to those for whom vaccination is recommended.

- Use antiviral agents according to available recommendations.

- Administer *Haemophilus influenzae* type B vaccine and pneumococcal conjugate and polysaccharide vaccines to those for whom they are recommended.

- Perform chest radiographs in persons suspected of having pneumonia and provide interpretations to treating clinicians.

- In persons with pneumonia, use appropriate diagnostic tests to determine the etiology.

- Follow existing guidelines for the treatment of pneumonia to target therapy toward the most likely pathogens, using the correct dose and duration of treatment.

---

## Future Directions

Much emphasis has been placed on preparing for the next influenza pandemic. Several steps for preventing resistant infections can be started in the early stages of a pandemic (table 2). During the pandemic, additional studies of secondary bacterial pneumonia will be important for determining the spectrum of etiologies, the role of resistant pathogens, and the best choices for empiric therapy.

## Acknowledgments

The authors gratefully acknowledge Jeffrey Hageman, Alicia Fry, and Carolyn Bridges for their careful reviews of this manuscript.

## References


1 Fry AM, Shay DK, Holman RC, Curns AT, Anderson LJ: Trends in hospitalizations for pneumonia among persons aged 65 years or older in the United States, 1988–2002. JAMA 2005;294:2712–2719.

2 Mandell GL, Bennett EJ, Dolin R (eds): Mandell, Douglas, and Bennett's principles and practice of infectious diseases, ed 6. San Diego, Elsevier/Churchill Livingstone, 2005.

3 Foy HM, Kenny GE, Cooney MK, Allan ID: Long-term epidemiology of infections with *Mycoplasma pneumoniae*. J Infect Dis 1979;139:681–687.

4 Grabowska K, Hogberg L, Penttinen P, Svensson A, Ekdahl K: Occurrence of invasive pneumococcal disease and number of excess cases due to influenza. BMC Infect Dis 2006;6:58.

5 Talbot TR, Poehling KA, Hartert TV, et al: Seasonality of invasive pneumococcal disease: temporal relation to documented influenza and respiratory syncytial viral circulation. Am J Med 2005;118:285–291.

6 Thompson WW, Shay DK, Weintraub E, et al: Influenza-associated hospitalizations in the United States. JAMA 2004;292:1333–1340.

7   Arnold KE, Leggiadro RJ, Breiman RF, et al: Risk factors for carriage of drug-resistant *Streptococcus pneumoniae* among children in Memphis, Tennessee (see comments). J Pediatr 1996;128:757–764.

8   Kuehnert MJ, Kruszon-Moran D, Hill HA, et al: Prevalence of *Staphylococcus aureus* nasal colonization in the United States, 2001–2002. J Infect Dis 2006;193:172–179.

9   Mandell LA: Antimicrobial resistance and treatment of community-acquired pneumonia. Clin Chest Med 2005;26:57–64.

10  Sangthawan P, Chantaratchada S, Chanthadisai N, Wattanathum A: Prevalence and clinical significance of community-acquired penicillin-resistant pneumococcal pneumonia in Thailand. Respirology 2003;8:208–212.

11  Song JH, Jung SI, Ki HK, et al: Clinical outcomes of pneumococcal pneumonia caused by antibiotic-resistant strains in Asian countries: a study by the Asian Network for Surveillance of Resistant Pathogens. Clin Infect Dis 2004;38:1570–1578.

12  Yu VL, Chiou CC, Feldman C, et al: An international prospective study of pneumococcal bacteremia: correlation with in vitro resistance, antibiotics administered, and clinical outcome. Clin Infect Dis 2003;37:230–237.

13  Bryan C, Talwani R, Stinson M: Penicillin dosing for pneumococcal pneumonia. Chest 1997;112:1657–1664.

14  Aspa J, Rajas O, Rodriguez de Castro F, et al: Drug-resistant pneumococcal pneumonia: clinical relevance and related factors. Clin Infect Dis 2004;38:787–798.

15  Aspa J, Rajas O, Rodriguez de Castro F, et al: Impact of initial antibiotic choice on mortality from pneumococcal pneumonia. Eur Respir J 2006;27:1010–1019.

16  Yu VL, Baddour LM: Infection by drug-resistant *Streptococcus pneumoniae* is not linked to increased mortality. Clin Infect Dis 2004;39:1086–1087.

17  Centers for Disease Control and Prevention: Effects of new penicillin susceptibility breakpoints for *Streptococcus pneumoniae*: United States, 2006–2007. MMWR Morb Mortal Wkly Rep 2008;57:1353–1355.

18  Sacho H, Klugman KP, Koornhof HJ, Ruff P: Community-acquired pneumonia in an adult due to a multiply-resistant pneumococcus. J Infect 1987;14:188–189.

19  Buckingham SC, McCullers JA, Lujan-Zilbermann J, Knapp KM, Orman KL, English BK: Early vancomycin therapy and adverse outcomes in children with pneumococcal meningitis. Pediatrics 2006;117:1688–1694.

20  Dowell SF, Smith T, Leversedge K, Snitzer J: Failure of treatment of pneumonia associated with highly resistant pneumococci in a child. Clin Infect Dis 1999;29:462–463.

21  Daum RS, Nachman JP, Leitch CD, Tenover FC: Nosocomial epiglottitis associated with penicillin- and cephalosporin-resistant *Streptococcus pneumoniae* bacteremia. J Clin Microbiol 1994;32:246–248.

22  Clinical and Laboratory Standards Institute: Performance standards for antimicrobial susceptibility testing: fifteenth informational supplement. Approved standard M100-S15. 2005.

23  Feikin DR, Schuchat A, Kolczak M, et al: Mortality from invasive pneumococcal pneumonia in the era of antibiotic resistance, 1995–1997. Am J Public Health 2000;90:223–229.

24  Pallares R, Capdevila O, Linares J, et al: The effect of cephalosporin resistance on mortality in adult patients with nonmeningeal systemic pneumococcal infections. Am J Med 2002;113:120–126.

25  Urban C, Rahman N, Zhao X, et al: Fluoroquinolone-resistant *Streptococcus pneumoniae* associated with levofloxacin therapy. J Infect Dis 2001;184:794–798.

26  Perez-Trallero E, Garcia-Arenzana JM, Jimenez JA, Peris A: Therapeutic failure and selection of resistance to quinolones in a case of pneumococcal pneumonia treated with ciprofloxacin. Eur J Clin Microbiol Infect Dis 1990;9:905–906.

27  Klugman KP: Bacteriological evidence of antibiotic failure in pneumococcal lower respiratory tract infections. Eur Respir J Suppl 2002;36:3s-8s.

28  Fuller JD, Low DE. A review of *Streptococcus pneumoniae* infection treatment failures associated with fluoroquinolone resistance. Clin Infect Dis 2005;41:118–121.

29  Moreno S, Garcia-Leoni ME, Cercenado E, Diaz MD, Bernaldo de Quiros JC, Bouza E: Infections caused by erythromycin-resistant *Streptococcus pneumoniae*: incidence, risk factors, and response to therapy in a prospective study. Clin Infect Dis 1995;20:1195–1200.

30  Daneman N, McGeer A, Green K, Low DE: Macrolide resistance in bacteremic pneumococcal disease: implications for patient management. Clin Infect Dis 2006;43:432–438.

31  Gopal V, Bisno AL, Silverblatt FJ: Failure of vancomycin treatment in *Staphylococcus aureus* endocarditis. In vivo and in vitro observations. JAMA 1976;236:1604–1606.

32  Chambers HF, Mills J, Drake TA, Sande MA: Failure of a once-daily regimen of cefonicid for treatment of endocarditis due to *Staphylococcus aureus*. Rev Infect Dis 1984;6(suppl 4):S870–S874.

33 Geiseler PJ, Rice TW, McCulley DJ, Lewis SM, Berzins BL: Failure of medical therapy in tricuspid endocarditis due to *Staphylococcus aureus*. Chemotherapy 1984;30:408–412.

34 Ruiz ME, Guerrero IC, Tuazon CU: Endocarditis caused by methicillin-resistant *Staphylococcus aureus*: treatment failure with linezolid. Clin Infect Dis 2002;35:1018–1020.

35 Hageman JC: Severe community-acquired pneumonia due to *Staphylococcus aureus*, 2003–04 influenza season. Emerg Infect Dis 2006;12:894–899.

36 Tseng MH, Wei BH, Lin WJ, et al: Fatal sepsis and necrotizing pneumonia in a child due to community-acquired methicillin-resistant *Staphylococcus aureus*: case report and literature review. Scand J Infect Dis 2005;37:504–507.

37 Torell E, Molin D, Tano E, Ehrenborg C, Ryden C: Community-acquired pneumonia and bacteraemia in a healthy young woman caused by methicillin-resistant *Staphylococcus aureus* (MRSA) carrying the genes encoding Panton-Valentine leukocidin (PVL). Scand J Infect Dis 2005;37:902–904.

38 Peleg AY, Munckhof WJ: Fatal necrotising pneumonia due to community-acquired methicillin-resistant *Staphylococcus aureus* (MRSA). Med J Aust 2004;181:228–229.

39 Garnier F, Tristan A, Francois B, et al: Pneumonia and new methicillin-resistant *Staphylococcus aureus* clone. Emerg Infect Dis 2006;12:498–500.

40 Frazee BW, Salz TO, Lambert L, Perdreau-Remington F: Fatal community-associated methicillin-resistant *Staphylococcus aureus* pneumonia in an immunocompetent young adult. Ann Emerg Med 2005;46:401–404.

41 Enayet I, Nazeri A, Johnson LB, Riederer K, Pawlak J, Saravolatz LD: Community-associated methicillin-resistant *Staphylococcus aureus* causing chronic pneumonia. Clin Infect Dis 2006;42:e57–e60.

42 Chua AP, Lee KH: Fatal bacteraemic pneumonia due to community-acquired methicillin-resistant *Staphylococcus aureus*. Singapore Med J 2006;47:546–548.

43 Labandeira-Rey M, Couzon F, Boisset S, et al: *Staphylococcus aureus* Panton-Valentine leukocidin causes necrotizing pneumonia. Science 2007;315:1130–1133.

44 Wunderink RG, Rello J, Cammarata SK, Croos-Dabrera RV, Kollef MH: Linezolid vs vancomycin: analysis of two double-blind studies of patients with methicillin-resistant *Staphylococcus aureus* nosocomial pneumonia. Chest 2003;124:1789–1797.

45 Hers JF, Masurel N, Mulder J: Bacteriology and histopathology of the respiratory tract and lungs in fatal Asian influenza. Lancet 1958;2:1141–1143.

46 Hinshaw V, Olsen C, Dybdahl-Sissoko N, Evans D: Apoptosis: a mechanism of cell killing by influenza A and B viruses. J Virol 1994;68:3667–3673.

47 Jakab GJ, Warr GA, Knight ME: Pulmonary and systemic defenses against challenge with Staphylococcus aureus in mice with pneumonia due to influenza A virus. J Infect Dis 1979;140:105–108.

48 McCullers JA, Rehg JE: Lethal synergism between influenza virus and *Streptococcus pneumoniae*: characterization of a mouse model and the role of platelet-activating factor receptor. J Infect Dis 2002;186:341–350.

49 Davison VE, Sanford BA: Factors influencing adherence of *Staphylococcus aureus* to influenza A virus-infected cell cultures. Infect Immun 1982;37:946–955.

50 McCullers JA, Bartmess KC: Role of neuraminidase in lethal synergism between influenza virus and *Streptococcus pneumoniae*. J Infect Dis 2003;187:1000–1009.

51 Thompson WW, Shay DK, Weintraub E, et al: Mortality associated with influenza and respiratory syncytial virus in the United States. JAMA 2003;289:179–186.

52 O'Brien KL, Walters MI, Sellman J, et al: Severe pneumococcal pneumonia in previously healthy children: the role of preceding influenza infection. Clin Infect Dis 2000;30:784–789.

53 Madhi SA, Klugman KP: A role for *Streptococcus pneumoniae* in virus-associated pneumonia. Nat Med 2004;10:811–813.

54 Francis JS, Doherty MC, Lopatin U, et al: Severe community-onset pneumonia in healthy adults caused by methicillin-resistant *Staphylococcus aureus* carrying the Panton-Valentine leukocidin genes. Clin Infect Dis 2005;40:100–107.

55 Brundage JF: Interactions between influenza and bacterial respiratory pathogens: implications for pandemic preparedness. Lancet Infect Dis 2006;6:303–312.

56 Taubenberger JK, Morens DM: 1918 Influenza: the mother of all pandemics. Emerg Infect Dis 2006;12:15–22.

57 Johnson NPAS, Mueller J: Updating the accounts: global mortality of the 1918–1920 'Spanish' influenza pandemic. Bull Hist Med 2002;76:105–115.

58 Taubenberger JK, Reid AH, Krafft AE, Bijwaard KE, Fanning TG: Initial genetic characterization of the 1918 'Spanish' influenza virus. Science 1997;275:1793–1796.

59 Tumpey TM, Garcia-Sastre A, Taubenberger JK, et al: Pathogenicity of influenza viruses with genes from the 1918 pandemic virus: functional roles of alveolar macrophages and neutrophils in limiting virus replication and mortality in mice. J Virol 2005;79:14933–14944.

60 Frost WH: Statistics of influenza morbidity (with special reference to certain factors in case incidence and case fatality). Public Health Reports 1920;35: 584–597.

61 Soper GA: The pandemic in the Army camps. JAMA 1918;72:1899–1909.

62 Stone WJ, Swift GW: Influenza and influenzal pneumonia at Fort Riley, Kansas (from September 15 to November 1, 1918). JAMA 1919;72:487–93.

63 Bloomfield A, Harrop GA: Clinical observations on epidemic influenza. Bull Johns Hopkins Hosp 1919; 30:1–9.

64 Smith W, Andrewes CH, Laidlaw PP: A virus obtained from influenza patients. Lancet 1933;225: 66–68.

65 Chickering HT, Park JH: *Staphylococcus aureus* pneumonia. JAMA 1919;72:617–623.

66 Petersdorf RG, Fusco JJ, Harter DH, Albrink WS: Pulmonary infections complicating Asian influenza. AMA Arch Intern Med 1959;103:262–272.

67 Robertson L, Caley JP, Moore J: Importance of *Staphylococcus aureus* in pneumonia in the 1957 epidemic of influenza A. Lancet 1958;2:233–236.

68 Martin C, Kunin C, Gottlieb L, Barnes M, Lieu C, Finland M: Asian Influenza A in Boston, 1957–58. I. Observations in thirty-two influenza-associated fatal cases. Arch Intern Med 1959;103:515–531.

69 Schwarzmann SW, Adler JL, Sullivan RJ Jr, Marine WM: Bacterial pneumonia during the Hong Kong influenza epidemic of 1968–1969. Arch Intern Med 1971;127:1037–1041.

70 Bisno AL, Griffin JP, Van Epps KA, Niell HB, Rytel MW: Pneumonia and Hong Kong influenza: a prospective study of the 1968–1969 epidemic. Am J Med Sci 1971;261:251–263.

71 Louria DB, Blumenfeld HL, Ellis JT, Kilbourne ED, Rogers DE: Studies on influenza in the pandemic of 1957–1958. II. Pulmonary complications of influenza. J Clin Invest 1959;38:213–265.

72 Marston BJ, Plouffe JF, File TM Jr, et al. Incidence of community-acquired pneumonia requiring hospitalization: results of a population-based active surveillance study in Ohio. The Community-Based Pneumonia Incidence Study Group. Arch Intern Med 1997;157:1709–1718.

73 Podewils LJ, Liedtke LA, McDonald LC, et al: A national survey of severe influenza-associated complications among children and adults, 2003–2004. Clin Infect Dis 2005;40:1693–1696.

74 Meltzer MI, Cox NJ, Fukuda K. The economic impact of pandemic influenza in the United States: priorities for intervention. Emerg Infect Dis 1999; 5:659–671.

75 Angeles Marcos M, Camps M, Pumarola T, et al: The role of viruses in the aetiology of community-acquired pneumonia in adults. Antivir Ther 2006; 11:351–359.

76 Creer DD, Dilworth JP, Gillespie SH, et al: Aetiological role of viral and bacterial infections in acute adult lower respiratory tract infection (LRTI) in primary care. Thorax 2006;61:75–79.

77 Oosterheert JJ, van Loon AM, Schuurman R, et al: Impact of rapid detection of viral and atypical bacterial pathogens by real-time polymerase chain reaction for patients with lower respiratory tract infection. Clin Infect Dis 2005;41:1438–1444.

78 Stralin K, Tornqvist E, Kaltoft MS, Olcen P, Holmberg H: Etiologic diagnosis of adult bacterial pneumonia by culture and PCR applied to respiratory tract samples. J Clin Microbiol 2006;44:643–645.

79 Peltola VT, Murti KG, McCullers JA: Influenza virus neuraminidase contributes to secondary bacterial pneumonia. J Infect Dis 2005;192:249–257.

80 Kaiser L, Wat C, Mills T, Mahoney P, Ward P, Hayden F: Impact of oseltamivir treatment on influenza-related lower respiratory tract complications and hospitalizations. Arch Intern Med 2003;163: 1667–1672.

81 McGeer A, Green KA, Plevneshi A, et al: Antiviral therapy and outcomes of influenza requiring hospitalization in Ontario, Canada. Clin Infect Dis 2007; 45:1568–1575.

82 Zangwill KM, Treanor JJ, Campbell JD, Noah DL, Ryea J: Evaluation of the safety and immunogenicity of a booster (third) dose of inactivated subvirion H5N1 influenza vaccine in humans. J Infect Dis 2008;197:580–583.

83 Nichol KL, Nordin JD, Nelson DB, Mullooly JP, Hak E: Effectiveness of influenza vaccine in the community-dwelling elderly. N Engl J Med 2007;357:1373–1381.

84 Kyaw MH, Rose CE, Jr., Fry AM, et al: The influence of chronic illnesses on the incidence of invasive pneumococcal disease in adults. J Infect Dis 2005; 192:377–386.

85 Yap FH, Ho PL, Lam KF, Chan PK, Cheng YH, Peiris JS: Excess hospital admissions for pneumonia, chronic obstructive pulmonary disease, and heart failure during influenza seasons in Hong Kong. J Med Virol 2004;73:617–623.

86 Couch RB: Influenza, influenza virus vaccine, and human immunodeficiency virus infection. Clin Infect Dis 1999;28:548–551.

87 Tasker SA, O'Brien WA, Treanor JJ, et al: Effects of influenza vaccination in HIV-infected adults: a double-blind, placebo-controlled trial. Vaccine 1998;16:1039–1042.

88  Lin JC, Nichol KL: Excess mortality due to pneumonia or influenza during influenza seasons among persons with acquired immunodeficiency syndrome. Arch Intern Med 2001;161:441–446.

89  Flannery B, Heffernan RT, Harrison LH, et al: Changes in invasive pneumococcal disease among HIV-infected adults living in the era of childhood pneumococcal immunization. Ann Intern Med 2006;144:1–9.

90  Fry AM, Facklam RR, Whitney CG, Plikaytis BD, Schuchat A: Multistate evaluation of invasive pneumococcal diseases in adults with human immunodeficiency virus infection: serotype and antimicrobial resistance patterns in the United States. J Infect Dis 2003;188:643–652.

91  Talbot TR, Hartert TV, Mitchel E, et al: Asthma as a risk factor for invasive pneumococcal disease. N Engl J Med 2005;352:2082–2090.

92  Asthma prevalence and control characteristics by race/ethnicity: United States, 2002. MMWR Morb Mortal Wkly Rep 2004;53:145–148.

93  Dobson R: US cigarette consumption falls to lowest point since 1951. BMJ 2006;332:687.

94  Adams W, Deaver K, Cochi S: Decline of childhood *Haemophilus influenza* type b (Hib) disease in the Hib vaccine era. J AMA 1993;269:221–226.

95  Whitney CG, Farley MM, Hadler J, et al: Increasing prevalence of multidrug-resistant *Streptococcus pneumoniae* in the United States. N Engl J Med 2000; 343:1917–1924.

96  Kyaw MH, Lynfield R, Schaffner W, et al: Effect of introduction of the pneumococcal conjugate vaccine on drug-resistant *Streptococcus pneumoniae*. N Engl J Med 2006;354:1455–1463.

97  Mandell LA, Wunderink RG, Anzueto A, et al: Infectious Diseases Society of America/American Thoracic Society consensus guidelines on the management of community-acquired pneumonia in adults. Clin Infect Dis 2007;44(suppl 2):S27–S72.

98  Bartlett JG: Diagnostic tests for etiologic agents of community-acquired pneumonia. Infect Dis Clin North Am 2004;18:809–827.

99  Chang NN, Murray CK, Houck PM, Bratzler DW, Greenway C, Guglielmo BJ: Blood culture and susceptibility results and allergy history do not influence fluoroquinolone use in the treatment of community-acquired pneumonia. Pharmacotherapy 2005;25:59–66.

100  Hopstaken RM, Butler CC, Muris JW, et al: Do clinical findings in lower respiratory tract infection help general practitioners prescribe antibiotics appropriately? An observational cohort study in general practice. Fam Pract 2006;23:180–187.

101  Speets AM, Hoes AW, van der Graaf Y, Kalmijn S, Sachs AP, Mali WP: CXR and pneumonia in primary care: diagnostic yield and consequences for patient management. Eur Respir J 2006;28:933–938.

102  Marrie TJ, Peeling RW, Fine MJ, Singer DE, Coley CM, Kapoor WN: Ambulatory patients with community-acquired pneumonia: the frequency of atypical agents and clinical course. Am J Med 1996; 101:508–515.

103  Christ-Crain M, Jaccard-Stolz D, Bingisser R, et al: Effect of procalcitonin-guided treatment on antibiotic use and outcome in lower respiratory tract infections: cluster-randomised, single-blinded intervention trial. Lancet 2004;363:600–607.

104  Madhi SA, Heera JR, Kuwanda L, Klugman KP: Use of procalcitonin and C-reactive protein to evaluate vaccine efficacy against pneumonia. PLoS Med 2005;2:e38.

105  Garcia Vazquez E, Mensa J, Martinez JA, et al: Lower mortality among patients with community-acquired pneumonia treated with a macrolide plus a beta-lactam agent versus a beta-lactam agent alone. Eur J Clin Microbiol Infect Dis 2005;24:190–195.

106  Baddour LM, Yu VL, Klugman KP, et al: Combination antibiotic therapy lowers mortality among severely ill patients with pneumococcal bacteremia. Am J Respir Crit Care Med 2004;170:440–444.

107  Barkai G, Greenberg D, Givon-Lavi N, Dreifuss E, Vardy D, Dagan R: Community prescribing and resistant *Streptococcus pneumoniae*. Emerg Infect Dis 2005;11:829–837.

108  Baquero F, Baquero-Artigao G, Canton R, Garcia-Rey C: Antibiotic consumption and resistance selection in *Streptococcus pneumoniae*. J Antimicrob Chemother 2002;50(suppl S2):27–37.

109  el Moussaoui R, de Borgie CA, van den Broek P, et al: Effectiveness of discontinuing antibiotic treatment after three days versus eight days in mild to moderate-severe community acquired pneumonia: randomised, double blind study. JAMA 2006;332: 1355.

110  Cole R. Problem. Kentucky Med J 1918:563–565.

111  Austrian R, Douglas RM, Schiffman G, et al: Prevention of pneumococcal pneumonia by vaccination. Trans Assoc Am Physicians 1976;89:184–194.

112  Dear K, Holden J, Andrews R, Tatham D. Vaccines for preventing pneumococcal infection in adults. Cochrane Database Syst Rev 2003:CD000422.

113  Butler JC, Breiman RF, Campbell JF, Lipman HB, Broome CV, Facklam RR: Pneumococcal polysaccharide vaccine efficacy: an evaluation of current recommendations. JAMA 1993;270:1826–1831.

114  Jackson LA, Neuzil KM, Yu O, et al: Effectiveness of pneumococcal polysaccharide vaccine in older adults. N Engl J Med 2003;348:1747–1755.

115 Shapiro ED, Clemens JD: A controlled evaluation of the protective efficacy of pneumococcal vaccine for patients at high risk of serious pneumococcal infections. Ann Intern Med 1984;101:325–330.

116 Facilitating influenza and pneumococcal vaccination through standing orders programs. MMWR Morb Mortal Wkly Rep 2003;52:68–69.

117 Thomas CM, Loewen A, Coffin C, Campbell NR: Improving rates of pneumococcal vaccination on discharge from a tertiary center medical teaching unit: a prospective intervention. BMC Public Health 2005;5:110.

118 Centers for Disease Control and Prevention: Direct and indirect effects of routine vaccination of children with 7-valent pneumococcal conjugate vaccine on incidence of invasive pneumococcal disease: United States, 1998–2003. MMWR Morb Mortal Wkly Rep 2005;54:893–897.

119 Dagan R, Sikuler-Cohen M, Zamir O, Janco J, Givon-Lavi N, Fraser D: Effect of a conjugate pneumococcal vaccine on the occurrence of respiratory infections and antibiotic use in day-care center attendees. Pediatr Infect Dis J 2001;20:951–958.

120 Centers for Disease Control and Prevention: Guidelines for preventing healthcare-associated pneumonia, 2003. MMWR Morbid Mort Wkly Report 2004;53:5–11.

121 Centers for Disease Control and Prevention: Guideline for hand hygiene in health-care settings: recommendations of the healthcare infection control practices advisory committee and the HICPAC/SHEA/APIC/IDSA hand hygiene task force. MMWR Morbid Mort Wkly Report 2002;51.

122 Hirsch EF, McKinney M: Epidemic of bronchopneumonia at Camp Grant, Ill. JAMA 1918;71:1735–1736.

123 Ely CF, Lloyd BJ, Hitchcock CD, Nickson DH: Influenza as seen at the Puget Sound Navy Yard. JAMA 1919;72:24–28.

124 Nuzum JW, Pilot I, Stangl FH, Bonar BE: Pandemic influenza and pneumonia in a large civilian hospital. JAMA 1918;71:1562–1565.

125 Blanton WB, Irons EE: A recent epidemic of acute respiratory infection at Camp Custer, Mich. JAMA 1918;71:1988–1991.

126 Brem WV, Bolling GE, Casper EJ: Pandemic influenza and secondary pneumonia at Camp Fremont, Calif. JAMA 1918;71:2138–2144.

127 Fry J: Influenza A (Asian) 1957:Clinical and epidemiological features in a general practice. BMJ 1958;2:259–261.

128 Hall JN, Stone MC, Simpson JC: The epidemic of pneumonia following influenza at Camp Logan, Texas. JAMA 1918;71:1986–1987.

129 Spooner LH, Scott LH, Heath EH: A bacteriologic study of the influenza epidemic at Camp Devens, Mass. JAMA 1919;72:155–159.

Matthew R. Moore, MD, MPH, Commander USPHS
Respiratory Diseases Branch, National Center for Immunization and Respiratory Diseases
Centers for Disease Control and Prevention
1600 Clifton Road, MS C-23, Atlanta, GA 30333 (USA)
Tel. +1 404 639 4887, Fax +1 404 639 3970, E-Mail matt.moore@cdc.hhs.gov

Weber JT (ed): Antimicrobial Resistance – Beyond the Breakpoint.
Issues Infect Dis. Basel, Karger, 2010, vol 6, pp 70–88

# Promoting Appropriate Antimicrobial Drug Use in the Outpatient Setting: What Works?

Edward A. Belongia[a] · Rita Mangione-Smith[b] · Mary Jo Knobloch[a]

[a]Marshfield Clinic Research Foundation, Marshfield, Wisc., and [b]Department of Pediatrics, University of Washington, Seattle, Wash., USA

## Abstract

Acute respiratory tract infections account for the majority of outpatient antimicrobial use, and physicians continue to prescribe these drugs inappropriately for cough, cold and flu symptoms despite lack of efficacy for viral illness. There have been modest reductions in antimicrobial prescribing for respiratory illness in recent years, but inappropriate use of broad-spectrum antimicrobials has increased. Multiple factors contribute to excessive and inappropriate antimicrobial prescribing, including patient expectations, time pressure and diagnostic uncertainty. Physicians perceive that patients will be more satisfied with an antimicrobial prescription, despite evidence that satisfaction with the physician and the office visit is largely determined by other factors. Market forces also contribute to excessive antimicrobial use in primary care.

Changing physician behavior is challenging, and traditional approaches, such as continuing medical education conferences and materials, have little impact. Evidence suggests that multifaceted interventions are more effective than single interventions, particularly if they involve personal or small group educational sessions ('academic detailing'). In general, it appears to be easier to influence decisions regarding the type of antimicrobial and duration of treatment as opposed to withholding antimicrobials entirely. Focusing patient communication on symptom alleviation can reduce patient opposition to non-antibiotic treatment recommendations and improve satisfaction. A contingency plan is helpful for patients who question non-antimicrobial treatment plans.

Appropriate antimicrobial use is increasingly viewed as a quality improvement issue, and performance measures have been established for pediatric upper respiratory infection and adult bronchitis. There is growing interest in pay for performance, but little is known regarding the relationship between physician reimbursement and appropriate antimicrobial prescribing. Clinical decision support tools are also promising but require further investigation. Over the next decade, we must acquire a better understanding of macro-level factors that contribute to inappropriate antimicrobial use, including social/cultural health beliefs and practices, physician reimbursement practices, pharmaceutical marketing, and organizational policies regarding return-to-work or child care following illness. Health care systems, pharmaceutical companies, medical schools, residency programs and managed care organizations must all take responsibility and work collaboratively to produce lasting change in antimicrobial prescribing habits.

In 1995, the writer Nicholas Wade predicted the day when the best medical advice would be: '(1) Don't get sick; (2) if you do, don't go to the hospital, and (3) if you must go to the hospital, don't take antibiotics.' [1]. The same advice is appropriate today for patients seen in the outpatient setting for acute respiratory illness. Multiple studies have demonstrated a strong and consistent link between antimicrobial use and the development of resistance at individual and population levels [2–7]. However, it is less clear how a reduction in outpatient antimicrobial use will affect the occurrence of resistant infections. The population dynamics of antimicrobial resistance are complex and poorly understood, but models of chromosomal or plasmid-mediated resistance in commensal flora suggest that resistance may persist as long as antimicrobial-resistant bacteria exist and individuals continue to receive antimicrobial treatment [8, 9]. The complete withdrawal of antimicrobial exposure might yield dramatic reductions in resistance over a period of years, but such a goal is not justifiable (or ethical) because there will always be patients with legitimate need for therapy. Despite these uncertainties, judicious use of antimicrobials may at least slow the spread of resistant pathogens, improve the quality of health care and help prevent adverse events.

Acute respiratory tract infections (ARIs) account for the majority of outpatient antimicrobial use, and many physicians prescribe these drugs inappropriately for cough, cold and flu symptoms despite their proven lack of efficacy for viral illness. A report by the Institute of Medicine in 1998 addressed this problem, noting that physicians and patients have not received adequate information about the appropriate use of antimicrobials and the risks of excessive use [10]. Multiple factors contribute to excessive and inappropriate antimicrobial prescribing for acute respiratory illness. Physicians and patients have different perceptions about antimicrobial use, and patient expectations influence physician prescribing behavior [11, 12]. It appears to be easier to influence decisions regarding antimicrobial selection and treatment duration than to persuade physicians to withhold antimicrobials entirely. Writing a prescription is a strategy to quickly end an office visit, an outcome that is important in an era of increasing patient volume and declining reimbursement. However, evidence indicates that the time savings are minimal, and that pediatric visits may even take longer when antimicrobials are prescribed [13–15]. Physicians perceive that patients will be more satisfied with an antimicrobial prescription, despite evidence that patient satisfaction is largely determined by factors other than receipt of an antimicrobial [16–18]. Diagnostic uncertainty also contributes to the pressure for antimicrobial use, since many ARIs are diagnosed and managed without laboratory confirmation, and the clinical manifestations of bacterial and viral infections often overlap. For example, duration of illness is often used as a surrogate marker for bacterial sinusitis, and adult guidelines support treatment of rhinosinusitis symptoms lasting more than 7 days with maxillary pain or tenderness [19]. Rhinovirus infections last a median of 9–11 days [20], and many patients receive antimicrobials unnecessarily based on the 7-day threshold.

Many physicians in outpatient practice have limited experience with severe manifestations of antimicrobial resistance, and may perceive the threat to be low [21]. These physicians may consider the balance between public health and individual patient care to be weighted more toward provision of antimicrobials for patients with an ARI, even when they recognize that the expected benefit is low. Past experience reinforces this behavior because many older practitioners acquired their antimicrobial prescribing habits during an era when resistance appeared to be a problem only in the hospital setting. Physician focus groups held by the Centers for Disease Control and Prevention (CDC) revealed the overarching sentiment that antimicrobial resistance was more of a national problem than a local problem [22]. Patient expectations (real or perceived) also tend to reinforce this behavior. Education is lacking among patients and the public, and there is little understanding of the difference between viral and bacterial infections [23–26].

Market forces also contribute to excessive antimicrobial use. Direct-to-consumer advertising is designed to promote antimicrobial selection based on taste, dosing interval and other factors unrelated to clinical efficacy. Pharmaceutical drug detailing emphasizes newer, broad-spectrum antimicrobials over generic, narrow-spectrum agents, and clinicians receive conflicting messages from marketing materials and practice guidelines [27].

Over the past decade, a variety of programs have been implemented at national, state and local levels to improve outpatient antimicrobial prescribing. Some have focused on educating or motivating clinicians to reduce antimicrobial use, others have focused on patient and public education, and several have developed multifaceted interventions that target clinicians, patients and the general public. Which of these approaches is most effective, and what can we recommend to the leaders of health care organizations and policy makers concerned about quality of care and rising health care costs? In this chapter, we discuss the impact of interventions to improve outpatient antimicrobial prescribing, identify gaps in knowledge, and suggest approaches for clinicians and health care organizations who want an evidence-based approach to appropriate antimicrobial use.

**Trends in Outpatient Antimicrobial Utilization**

In the United States, inappropriate antimicrobial prescribing rates peaked in the 1990s and declined modestly by the end of the decade. Data from the National Ambulatory Medical Care Survey indicate that antimicrobial use declined for ARIs during this time frame, but use of broad-spectrum antimicrobials increased dramatically in both children and adults [28, 29]. Overall antimicrobial use declined among both white and black children, but prescribing rates were consistently higher in whites [30]. Prescribing rates declined in the United States at both the population level and at the level of visits for ARI [31]. At the population level, reductions in prescribing rates may be due to a combination of reduced health care-seeking behavior (self care for illnesses recognized to be viral or limited access to care for those without medical insurance) and reduced prescribing by physicians when a visit does occur. Similar trends have been observed using claims data from 9 large health plans. From 1996 to 2000, prescribing rates for children aged between 3 months and less than 6 years declined approximately 25%, and reduced prescribing for otitis media accounted for nearly two-thirds of the total decrease [32].

Inappropriate use of broad-spectrum antimicrobials continues to be a problem, generating additional selection pressure for antimicrobial resistance in community-acquired pathogens. From 1996 to 2000, pediatric use of second-generation macrolide drugs (azithromycin, clarithromycin) increased dramatically in 9 large health plans, although they accounted for less than 10% of all antimicrobials dispensed [33]. From 1995 to 2002, fluoroquinolone prescribing for adults increased more than 300%, and over 40% of fluoroquinolone prescriptions were for diagnoses such as acute bronchitis, otitis media and acute upper respiratory infections [34]. These results emphasize the continued need for education and behavior change despite modest improvements in overall antimicrobial prescribing rates.

## Interventions to Improve Outpatient Antimicrobial Use

Changing physician behavior is challenging, and traditional approaches such as continuing medical education conferences and materials have little impact [35, 36]. The problem is especially complex in the case of antimicrobial prescribing, since behavior changes must occur among physicians and, to some extent, among patients as well. There is no single intervention or approach that is universally successful, but multifaceted interventions are more effective than single interventions, particularly if they involve personal or small group educational sessions (aka 'academic detailing') [37–39].

Table 1 summarizes 9 controlled studies that evaluated multifaceted interventions for patients, the public and physicians to reduce outpatient antimicrobial prescribing. Additional studies have evaluated educational interventions using only historical data for comparison, but the lack of a concurrent control group limits the interpretation of results, especially when the background rate of antimicrobial prescribing is known to be changing. All 9 studies shown in table 1 employed a concurrent control group, and some included multiple intervention arms. Clinician interventions included various combinations of academic detailing, performance feedback, expert presentations, guideline distribution, mailings and provision of patient education materials (pamphlets and posters). Patient and public interventions were based on CDC pamphlets and posters, locally developed educational materials, news media coverage and paid advertisements.

Outcomes for these studies are shown in table 2. The specific measures cannot be directly compared, but most were based on antimicrobial prescribing rates at the

**Table 1.** Controlled studies with multifaceted clinician and patient/public interventions to reduce outpatient antibiotic utilization.

| First author, year | Study design | Population/setting | Clinician interventions | Patient/public interventions |
|---|---|---|---|---|
| Belongia, 2001 [25] | CBA | 185 physicians and parents in rural communities of northern Wisconsin (USA) | Large and small group meetings for clinicians; printed materials based on CDC principles of appropriate antibiotic use | CDC pamphlets and posters distributed to parents, childcare providers, schools, community organizations and clinics |
| Belongia, 2005 [44] | CBA | Statewide program targeting primary care physicians, parents and the public in Wisconsin (USA) | Printed materials mailed to physicians annually; distribution of academic detailing packets and annual pneumococcal susceptibility report; multiple grand rounds and conference presentations; distribution of CD-ROM slide presentation and clinical practice fact sheets; resource binder for health plans; 2 satellite broadcasts by national experts | Mailings to childcare providers; distribution of pamphlets and posters to pharmacies and clinics; costumed characters at health fairs and community events; radio and television advertisements; newspaper and television coverage |
| Doyne, 2004 [75] | RCT | 11 pediatric practice groups in area of Cincinnati (Ohio, USA) | Presentation by CDC expert to local opinion leaders; academic detailing; distribution of locally developed practice guidelines | Parent focus groups; CDC pamphlets, posters and flyers distributed to clinics |
| Finkelstein, 2001 [32] | RCT | 12 pediatric practice groups affiliated with 2 managed care organizations | Small group educational sessions by 'peer leader'; follow-up visit and performance feedback 4 months later; printed materials provided to clinics and pamphlets mailed to parents | CDC pamphlet and cover letter mailed to families; pamphlets and posters distributed to clinics |
| Gonzales, 1999 [17] | CBA | 4 health maintenance organization group practices in Denver (Colo., USA) | Full intervention site received feedback of site-specific prescribing rates for acute bronchitis; small group academic detailing to review management of bronchitis with clinicians | Cover letter and educational materials mailed to households; pamphlets and posters distributed to clinic exam rooms and waiting areas |
| Hennessy, 2002 [76] | CBA | Physicians, health aides, residents in 13 Alaskan villages (3 regions) | Workshops for community health aides and physicians with follow-up visits. | Materials distributed in village-wide meetings, community fairs and high-school classrooms; newsletters sent to households |



Belongia · Mangione-Smith · Knobloch

**Table 1.** Continued

| First author, year | Study design | Population/setting | Clinician interventions | Patient/public interventions |
|---|---|---|---|---|
| Mainous, 2000 [23] | RCT | Primary care physicians providing Medicaid services to children in Kentucky (USA) | Intervention physicians randomized to receive either performance feedback only, patient education material only, or both. | CDC pamphlets mailed to physicians for patient education |
| Perz, 2002 [77] | CBA | Children enrolled in Medicaid in 4 counties of Tennesse (USA) | Clinician lectures, guideline distribution, physician newsletter, pamphlets distributed to parents and clinics | CDC pamphlets distributed to hospitals, clinics, dental offices, pharmacies, and parents of children in day care and grades K to 3 (5–9 years old); patient education materials provided to clinics |
| Welschen, 2004 [18] | RCT | 100 general practitioners in Utrecht (the Netherlands) | Group education meetings with consensus development; communication skills training; audit and feedback of prescribing behavior; meeting with physician assistants and pharmacists | Brochure and poster provided to waiting rooms, pharmacies and municipal health services |

CBA = Cost-benefit analysis; RCT = randomized controlled trial.

population, provider or visit level. One study evaluated an intervention to reduce antimicrobial utilization for acute bronchitis [40], but the others addressed overall prescribing for acute respiratory illness. In 7 studies, prescribing measures improved over time in both the intervention and control groups, consistent with the secular trend of declining antimicrobial use. The intervention-attributable effect was modest overall, and it exceeded 20% in only 1 study. This was a clinic-randomized intervention to improve prescribing for adult bronchitis [40] in a managed care setting. Eight studies reported a crude intervention-attributable effect in the range of 0–10%.

Little is known about the relationship between physician reimbursement and antimicrobial prescribing. One study suggested that fee-for-service reimbursement prompts physicians to prescribe more antimicrobials [41], but the impact of financial incentives has not been evaluated using controlled studies. An uncontrolled before-after study in Rochester (N.Y., USA) evaluated an intervention that included academic detailing, performance feedback and financial incentives to improve management of acute sinusitis [42]. The financial incentive was based on a scoring system related to patient satisfaction (20%), efficiency (40%) and quality (40%). Up to half of the quality component was based on compliance with an acute sinusitis care pathway that

**Table 2.** Outcomes of controlled studies with multifaceted clinician and patient/public interventions to reduce outpatient antibiotic utilization.

| First author, year | Comparison group | Major outcome measure | Intervention-attributable effect | Comment |
|---|---|---|---|---|
| Belongia, 2001 [25] | 1 control community (52 physicians) | Antibiotic prescriptions per clinician (reported separately for solid and liquid) | Solid: 11% (–19% change in intervention group vs. –8% change in control) Liquid: 23% (–11% in intervention vs. +12% in control) | No effect on carriage of penicillin-nonsusceptible *S. pneumoniae* in children attending day care |
| Belongia, 2005 [44] | Wisconsin vs. Minnesota (USA) | Mean number of antibiotic prescriptions per physician per year | 0% (–20% change in both Wisconsin and Minnesota from 1998–2003) | Retail sales of antimicrobial drugs (grams per capita) declined to a similar degree in Wisconsin and Minnesota. |
| Doyne, 2004 [75] | 6 control practices | Ratio of antibiotic prescriptions filled to number of office visits | 4% (–18% change in intervention group vs. –14% in control) | Academic detailing not effective |
| Finkelstein, 2001 [32] | 6 control practices | Antibiotic courses (based on pharmacy claims data) dispensed per person-year, reported separately for children aged 3–35 months and 36–71 months | Age 3–35 months: 7% –19% change in intervention group and –12% in control) Age 36–71 months: 10% (–15% in intervention group and –10% in control) | Adjusted intervention effect was 16% in younger group and 12% in older group after controlling for age, baseline prescribing and clustering by practice |
| Gonzales, 1999 [17] | 1 control clinic and 1 limited intervention clinic (patient education only) | % of incident acute bronchitis visits with antibiotic prescription | 24% (–26% for full intervention site vs. –2% control) | Limited intervention (patient education only) had no impact on antibiotic prescribing |
| Hennessy, 2002 [76] | 2,030 residents in control villages | Antibiotic courses per respiratory infection visit | 12% (–17% change in intervention group vs. –5% in control) | No effect on carriage of penicillin-nonsusceptible *S. pneumoniae* |
| Mainous, 2000 [23] | 62 physicians | % of ARI visits with antibiotic prescription | Education + feedback group: 7% (+15% change in intervention vs. +22% in control) | Antibiotic prescribing for ARI increased in all groups after intervention; education + feedback was similar to education alone or feedback alone |

| First author, year | Comparison group | Major outcome measure | Intervention-attributable effect | Comment |
|---|---|---|---|---|
| Perz, 2002 [77] | 3 urban counties | Antibiotic prescriptions per 100 person-years | 11% (–19% change in intervention county vs. –8% in control counties) | Prescribing reduction was greatest for children 1–4 years old |
| Welschen, 2004 [18] | 47 general practitioners | % of ARI visits with antibiotic prescription | 12% (–4% intervention vs. +8% control) | Patient satisfaction was not affected by intervention |

included initial symptomatic therapy, selection of amoxicillin as first-line antimicrobial treatment, and absence of imaging studies for uncomplicated sinusitis. Physicians scoring above the 95th percentile for the group received a 5% rebate in capitation withhold (a payment mechanism for physicians in the United States), and those in the 5th percentile or below were penalized by an additional 10% withhold. Deviations from the recommended care pathway declined 20% after this intervention, but most improvements in antimicrobial use were based on selection of appropriate first-line agents rather than volume of antimicrobials prescribed.

The effects of antimicrobial prescribing interventions at the state, regional or national level are poorly understood. In Canada, a change in reimbursement guidelines for fluoroquinolone use in elderly adults provided an opportunity to study the impact of regulatory changes at the provincial level [43]. In 1997, Nova Scotia implemented new requirements for additional paperwork with each fluoroquinolone prescription. Prescribers were required to document that the drug was being prescribed for a guideline-approved use, and this documentation had to accompany the prescription. Data from the provincial drug claim database demonstrated that fluoroquinolone prescriptions in older adults declined from 20 to 4% of antimicrobial prescriptions, a relative decrease of 80%. The decline occurred immediately, although the total number of antimicrobial prescriptions remained stable.

In Wisconsin (USA), a 5-year multifaceted campaign for primary care clinicians and the general public was associated with a 20% reduction in antimicrobial prescribing rates, but this was identical to the decline in a comparison state (Minnesota) over the same time period, despite the relative absence of specific educational interventions in Minnesota [44].

Several studies have evaluated strategies to improve selection of appropriate first-line drugs or duration of treatment. One of the earliest interventions compared a mailed brochure with personal visits (academic detailing) to reduce prescribing of oral cephalosporins among Tennessee (USA) physicians with high prescribing rates [45]. The visits were conducted by a project pharmacist in one arm, and by a physician in the other arm. The mailed brochure had no impact on prescribing, and the drug educator visits had a modest effect. However, substantial reductions in cephalosporin use were observed in physicians who received an academic detailing visit from another physician, with an attributable intervention effect of 21% for the average number of patients receiving cephalosporins.

A randomized controlled trial (RCT) was conducted to improve compliance with pharyngitis treatment recommendations in a group of 182 general practitioners in Victoria (Australia) [46]. The intervention included an educational mailing and academic detailing visits by the project pharmacist. Physicians were encouraged to use narrow spectrum antimicrobials (penicillin V, erythromycin) for tonsillitis. Compliance with the guidelines improved in both the intervention and control groups, but the improvement in the intervention group was significantly greater than that in the control group. In Ontario (Canada), a RCT evaluated performance feedback on antimicrobial prescribing along with mailed educational bulletins to encourage use of narrow-spectrum, first-line antimicrobials in a group of 250 physicians [47]. The impact was minimal: the proportion of visits involving a first-line antimicrobial increased by 2.6% in the intervention group and declined 1.7% in the control group.

In Finland, a longitudinal study was conducted to evaluate guideline compliance for 6 major infections (otitis media, sinusitis, pharyngitis, acute bronchitis, urinary tract infection, bacterial skin infection) [48]. Thirty Finnish health care centers participated in a 'train the trainer' program that provided a multifaceted educational program for one physician from each center. Adherence to prescribing guidelines was a primary outcome measure, and a secondary outcome was the proportion of patients receiving antimicrobials by indication. The intervention generated significant improvements in appropriate use of first-line antimicrobial agents for sinusitis, acute bronchitis, and urinary tract infection. Unfortunately, there was no improvement in the proportion of patients receiving inappropriate antimicrobial therapy for upper respiratory infection, acute bronchitis or viral pharyngitis. Physicians in a group of 20 control health centers, which did not participate in the 'train-the-trainer' program, adhered to the prescribing guidelines about as well as physicians from the intervention health care centers. Overall, these results suggest that adherence to treatment guidelines may be easier to achieve than an overall reduction in inappropriate antimicrobial use.

## Clinical Decision Support to Improve Antimicrobial Prescribing

There is growing interest in clinical decision support to improve quality of care, but much of the research has focused on inpatient care issues. Efforts to implement and evaluate decision support tools for outpatient antimicrobial use have been limited. In rural Utah (USA), a 2-year community randomized trial compared two different strategies to improve antimicrobial use for outpatient respiratory infections [49]. One arm of the trial received a community intervention alone, and the other arm received both a community intervention and a direct intervention with clinicians. The latter was based on decision-support tools delivered either on paper or via a personal digital assistant (PDA). Twelve study communities were randomly assigned to one of these arms, and 6 additional communities served as non-study controls. The PDA-based decision support tool generated diagnostic and therapeutic recommendations after the physician entered data on the suspected diagnosis and specific signs/symptoms. The decision support tools were introduced in small group meetings, and local opinion leaders served as champions. Physicians were asked to use the decision support tools for 200 consecutive patients with acute respiratory illness, and antimicrobial prescribing rates were compared across groups.

During the first intervention year, there was no significant change in antimicrobial prescribing in any of the study arms. However, prescribing rates (based on IMS Health data) declined 10% from baseline during the second year in the decision support communities, while the prescribing rates increased by 6% in the non-study communities and 1% in the education-only communities. The difference between the decision support communities and the education-only communities was statistically significant. The analysis based on medical record review demonstrated that the decision support intervention yielded an 11% absolute reduction in antimicrobial prescribing for diagnoses where antimicrobials are not indicated, compared to a 2% absolute reduction in the education-only communities.

A point-of-care decision support tool was used to improve antimicrobial selection and duration of therapy for acute otitis media [50]. This was a RCT involving 38 resident and attending physicians at a university-affiliated primary care pediatrics clinic in Seattle (Wash., USA) In this setting computerized prescriptions were used, and providers in the intervention arm received pop-up windows with evidence-based recommendations related to their antimicrobial selection, indication and duration of treatment. Providers had the option to view more detailed information or an abstract of the publication that was the source of the recommendation. The primary outcome was a reduction in duration of therapy below 10 days; a secondary outcome was a reduction in use of any antimicrobial for otitis media. The proportion of episodes treated with less than 10 days of antimicrobials increased by 44% in the intervention group and 10% in the control group (p < 0.01). The proportion receiving any antimicrobial increased 17% in the control group and 4% in the intervention group, but the difference across groups was of borderline significance.

## Health Plan Performance Measures to Promote Improved Prescribing

One mechanism for underscoring the importance of specific medical practices is the public reporting of performance on selected quality of care measures. The most widely used system of performance measures, the Healthcare Effectiveness Data and Information Set (HEDIS)®, allows for measurement of the degree to which evidence-based medical practices are being implemented, allows purchasers and consumers to select health plans based on such information, and raises general awareness of the need to improve on measured practices.

The CDC collaborated with the National Committee for Quality Assurance in 2001 to develop 2 HEDIS performance measures focused on antimicrobial use in the pediatric population. The first measure focuses on antimicrobial prescribing rates for upper respiratory infection and the second assesses the frequency of laboratory testing (for group A *Streptococcus*) in children who receive antimicrobials for pharyngitis. In 2005, 70% of commercially insured children who received antimicrobials for pharyngitis were also tested for Group A *Streptococcus*; the proportion was only 52% among those receiving services from Medicaid (the heath care program for people with low incomes in the United States) [51].

In 2004, the National Committee for Quality Assurance launched a second measure development process in conjunction with the Coalition for Affordable Healthcare Quality and the CDC. This measure examines antimicrobial prescribing for adults diagnosed with acute bronchitis. The first year of reporting demonstrated that antimicrobial use for acute bronchitis remains unacceptably high. Among patients 18–64 years old, 66% (commercial insurance) and 69% (Medicaid) received an antimicrobial prescription within 3 days after a diagnosis of acute bronchitis.


**AHRQ Analysis of Quality Improvement Strategies for Antimicrobial Prescribing**

In 2006, the Agency for Healthcare Research and Quality (AHRQ) published a report on antimicrobial prescribing as a quality improvement measure (www.ahrq.gov/clinic/tp/medigaptp.htm). This report, prepared by investigators at the Stanford-UCSF Evidence-Based Practice Center, systematically examined the effects of quality improvement strategies for reducing inappropriate outpatient antimicrobial use, and for reducing inappropriate selection of broad-spectrum agents when narrow-spectrum agents are indicated. The authors reviewed RCTs, controlled before-after studies, and interrupted time series studies on the decision to use antimicrobials. The primary outcomes were either the proportion of patients receiving any antimicrobial, or the proportion receiving a drug that was in accordance with recommended first-line therapy. Two reviewers independently abstracted data on interventions, study populations, targets and outcomes. The different quality improvement strategies were compared based on the median effect for the primary outcomes.

Fifty-four studies met the inclusion criteria, including 34 studies addressing the decision to prescribe antimicrobials and 26 studies focusing on selection of the appropriate agent (6 studies addressed both issues). The authors concluded that the methodologic quality of the included studies was generally fair. Most trials were classified as RCTs, but often failed to describe the theoretical basis for interventions. The investigators reported the following conclusions from this analysis:

1 Quality improvement strategies are moderately effective at reducing the inappropriate prescribing of antimicrobials and improving the appropriate selection of antimicrobials. The median absolute reduction in antimicrobial use was only 8.9% (interquartile range 6.7–12.4%) in the reviewed studies. For studies targeting selection of the appropriate agent, the median absolute reduction was 10.6% (interquartile range 3.4–18.2%).

2 Although no single quality improvement strategy is clearly superior, active clinician education may be more effective in certain settings. There was no single intervention or group of interventions that was highly effective. Active educational interventions appeared to be more effective in studies focusing on the decision to prescribe antimicrobials, but the difference was not significant. Surprisingly, clinician education alone appeared to be less effective than clinician education plus audit and feedback of prescribing behavior for those studies that focused on selection of the appropriate drug.

3 Interventions targeting prescribing for all acute respiratory tract infections may exert a greater effect on overall prescribing than interventions targeting specific types of acute respiratory infections. The authors extrapolated antimicrobial prescribing data to the population level when possible for each study, and they found that interventions focused on all ARIs, rather than specific diagnoses, had the greatest potential impact on antimicrobial use. Interventions focused on particular diagnoses (such as sinusitis or pharyngitis) tended to have greater effect sizes at the individual level, but the population-level effects were more modest.

4 Study design and quality should be improved. Studies that formally evaluate the cost effectiveness of interventions to improve antimicrobial treatment and selection are needed, and studies should evaluate the potential harm of such interventions. A substantial number of studies suffered from methodologic limitations, such as lack of randomization and failure to document whether the educational interventions were received by the participants. Multifaceted intervention studies generally require analysis at the level of the clinic, population, or geographic area (such as a city or county). Randomized studies at the clinic level are feasible and have proven useful for evaluation of antimicrobial prescribing interventions. However, randomization is often impossible at the level of communities, counties, or other large geographic areas due to cost considerations and limited number of units available for allocation. In addition, delivery of interventions is more complex and difficult to measure in larger populations. As a result, non-randomized studies have predominated despite the methodologic superiority of group randomized trials.

When physicians perceive that a patient or parent expects an antimicrobial they are significantly more likely to inappropriately prescribe [12, 16, 52–57]. However, physician perceptions are poorly correlated with actual patient or parent expectations for antimicrobials [16, 53–55, 58, 59]. Although 50–70% of patients and parents expect to receive antimicrobials when they attend visits for ARI, only 1–6% make direct verbal requests for them [58, 60]. Even when no direct requests for antimicrobials are made, physicians still perceive an expectation 34% of the time [58]. If miscommunication about expectations could be avoided, much inappropriate antimicrobial prescribing could potentially be prevented.

In pediatrics, physician perceptions are largely predicted by various indirect parent communication behaviors that occur during visits for ARI [57]. Through a series of qualitative studies, Stivers [61–63] identified 3 parent communication practices that appeared to be related to physician perceptions that parents expected antimicrobials. These were the parent suggesting a candidate diagnosis early in the visit, resisting the physician's diagnosis in viral cases, and resisting the physician's non-antimicrobial treatment plans [61–63]. Presenting a candidate diagnosis involves the parent suggesting their child has a diagnosis where antimicrobials are commonly prescribed, for example 'I think he's got sinusitis again,' rather then just listing their child's symptoms, 'She has a cough and a runny nose'. Diagnosis resistance occurs when the parent questions the physician's diagnosis. Treatment resistance is when the parent questions the physician's treatment plan. Confirming what Stivers hypothesized based on qualitative analyses, a recent quantitative study showed that parents who use candidate diagnoses are significantly more likely to expect antimicrobials (27% increase) and be perceived as expecting them (9% increase) [64]. Surprisingly, parents who expect antimicrobials are no more likely to question their child's physician about non-antimicrobial treatment plans than parents without expectations. Whether parents expect antimicrobials or not, they are significantly more likely to be perceived as expecting antimicrobials (20% increase) when they question the physician's treatment plan [64]. These findings may explain some of the gap between actual and perceived expectations.

Parent questioning of non-antimicrobial treatment plans is largely determined by how physicians present these plans to them. Stivers identified 2 main ways that physicians present non-antimicrobial treatment plans during visits for ARI: positively formatted treatment plans (e.g. 'You can try running a humidifier in her room at night to settle the cough down') and negatively formatted or 'rule-out' treatment plans (e.g. 'An antibiotic isn't going to touch this thing') [63]. When physicians use negatively formatted treatment plans and rule-out the need for antimicrobials, parents are significantly more likely to question the plan (24% increase) [64]. Thus, focusing treatment plans on what parents can do to make their child feel better rather then on why antimicrobials are unnecessary decreases parent questioning of treatment plans and may decrease inappropriate antimicrobial prescribing that results from physicians perceiving pressure to prescribe.

Although much of the work examining the relationship between communication practices and inappropriate antimicrobial prescribing has been conducted in the pediatric setting, many of the findings apply to the adult medical setting as well [60]. Adult patients similarly employ candidate diagnoses to indirectly communicate their expectations for antimicrobials, but also use additional communication practices in this regard. Scott et al. [60] found adults most frequently portray their illness as being severe and thus in need of treatment beyond what they have tried at home, for example 'I just can't shake it, Doc'. They also appeal to non-medical circumstances such as going out of town on a vacation, or noting that the last time they had this illness another physician in the same office treated with an antimicrobial and it seemed to work.

*Communication, Satisfaction and Antimicrobial Prescribing*

Contrary to commonly held beliefs among medical professionals, providing an antimicrobial prescription is unlikely to result in a satisfied patient or parent in the absence of high-quality communication [11, 65]. In visits for ARI, parent satisfaction is most strongly related to the quality of communication during the visit, rather than unfulfilled expectations for antimicrobials [11, 56]. Among parents who don't receive expected antimicrobials, those offered a contingency plan from the physician (i.e. the possibility of receiving antimicrobials in the future if their child does not get better) have a higher mean satisfaction score than parents not receiving a contingency plan (76 vs. 59% on a 0–100% scale; $p < 0.05$) [58]. Parents who receive a contingency plan also trend toward having higher mean satisfaction than parents who receive antimicrobials (76 vs. 65%; $p = 0.07$). This suggests that physicians should consider providing a contingency plan to parents who question non-antimicrobial treatment plans as it may preserve or enhance their satisfaction with the visit and prevent inappropriate antimicrobial prescribing.

Among adult patients, satisfaction similarly is not related to receiving expected antimicrobials [16, 55]. Rather, it is strongly associated with how well physicians explain things during the visit and how much time they spend with the patient.

*Communication-Based Interventions to Decrease Inappropriate Antimicrobial Prescribing*

Data on the effectiveness of communication-based interventions aimed at decreasing inappropriate antimicrobial prescribing are sparse. One multi-faceted intervention trial included a communication skills training session for physicians [66]. The

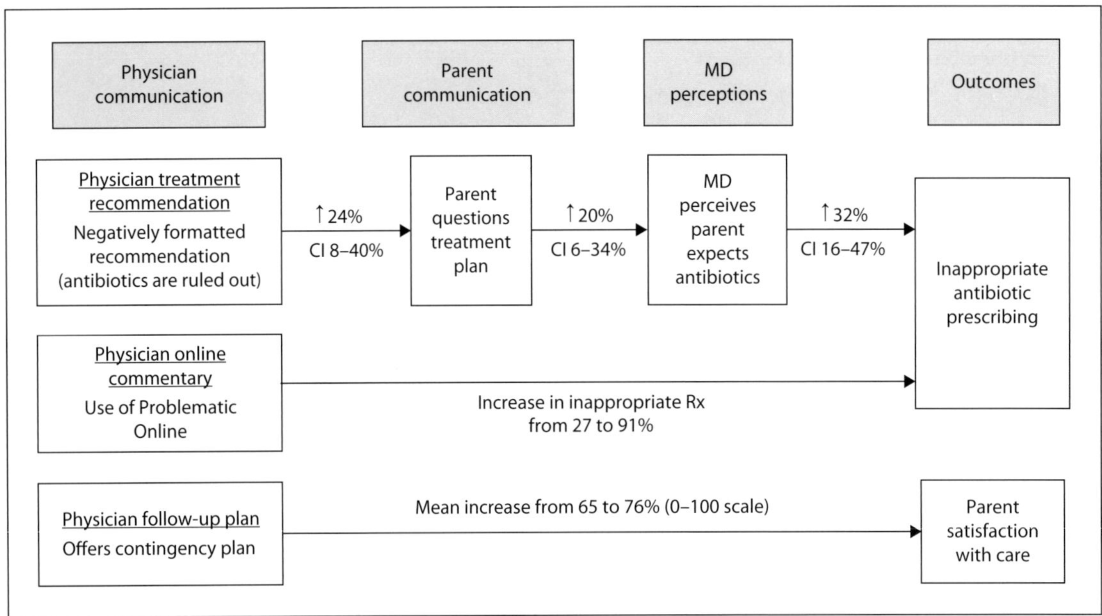


**Fig. 1.** The relationships between physician-parent communication, physician perceptions, inappropriate antimicrobial prescribing and satisfaction.

communication skills included exploring patient worries and expectations, and informing patients about the natural course of symptoms, self-medication and alarm symptoms that indicated the need for a return visit. Although physicians in the treatment arm significantly reduced their rates of inappropriate antimicrobial prescribing, it is difficult to know how much of this improvement was attributable to the communication training they received as opposed to other interventions employed, such as small group meetings and performance feedback.

The relationships between doctor-patient (or doctor-parent) communication, inappropriate prescribing and satisfaction are complex. Figure 1 represents a summary of research findings to date and suggests some key leverage points for future interventions aimed at improving communication during medical encounters for ARI. As shown in the figure, a communication practice called 'online commentary' shows promise for potentially decreasing rates of inappropriate antimicrobial prescribing [67]. This physician communication practice consists of describing what is being seen, felt or heard during the physical examination of the patient. The 2 primary types of online commentary are: (1) online commentary suggesting a problem on physical examination ('problem' online commentary), for example 'That cough sounds very chesty', and (2) online commentary that indicates the physical examination findings are not problematic ('no problem' online commentary), for example 'Her throat is only slightly red'.

In one study, antimicrobials were prescribed 91% of the time in cases where the presumed diagnosis was viral and the physician used at least some 'problem' online commentary. In contrast, when physicians exclusively used 'no problem' online commentary in such cases, antimicrobials were prescribed only 27% of the time. Use of 'no problem' online commentary did not add significantly to visit length [68]. Thus 'no problem' online commentary is a communication technique that may provide an effective and efficient method for resisting perceived pressure to prescribe antimicrobials.

Physician-patient/parent communication is clearly associated with inappropriate antimicrobial prescribing. Future interventions must continue to address these communication issues if we are to make further progress in addressing this serious public health problem.


**Future Directions**

The impact of educational interventions on appropriate antimicrobial prescribing has been modest at best, and the sustainability of intervention effects is largely unknown. Research to date has not identified any single intervention that will substantially reduce antimicrobial prescribing in all clinical settings. Factors limiting the generalizability of results include poorly defined targets for prescribing, variation in geographic scope of interventions, organizational priorities and limited funding. Well-designed, RCTs are needed to evaluate novel approaches to improve outpatient antimicrobial utilization, including economic incentives and formulary restrictions. These interventions must substantially reduce antimicrobial prescribing for viral illness without limiting appropriate antimicrobial use for bacterial infections. Such a goal is justified as a quality of care measure even if the impact on resistant infections is uncertain.

We must acquire a better understanding of macro-level factors that contribute to inappropriate antimicrobial use, including social/cultural health beliefs and practices, pharmaceutical marketing, and organizational policies such as return-to-work, return-to-school and child care attendance [27, 69, 70]. In addition, pharmaceutical companies, health care systems, medical schools, residency programs and managed care organizations must all work collaboratively to produce lasting change in antimicrobial prescribing habits.

Reframing antimicrobial prescribing as quality initiatives (e.g. HEDIS measures) may motivate managed care organizations to monitor prescribing rates and promote careful antimicrobial use through educational and policy interventions. In particular, the combination of educational strategies with organizational policies, formularies and antimicrobial stewardship programs may promote appropriate antimicrobial utilization [71–74]. There will be an ongoing need for education, promotion of appropriate vaccination and institutional infection-control practices as important components of the long-term effort to combat antimicrobial resistance.

**References**

1   Wade N: Pax antibiotica. New York Times Magazine, Oct 15, 1995.
2   Arason V, Kristinsson K, Sigurdsson J, Stefansdottir G, Molstad S, Gudmundsson S: Do antimicrobials increase the carriage rate of penicillin-resistant pneumococci in children? Cross-sectional prevalence study. Br Med J 1996;313:387–391.
3   Albrich W, Monnet D, Harbarth S: Antibiotic selection pressure and resistance in *Streptococcus pneumoniae* and *Streptococcus pyogenes*. Emerg Infect Dis 2004;10:514–517.
4   Ho PL, Tse WS, Tsang KWT, Kwok TK, Ng TK, Cheng VCC, et al: Risk factors for acquisition of levofloxacin-resistant *Streptococcus pneumoniae*: a case-control study. Clin Infect Dis 2001;32:701–707.
5   Nava JM, Bella F, Garau J, Lite J, Morera MA, Marti C, et al: Predictive factors for invasive disease due to penicillin-resistant *Streptococcus pneumoniae*: a population-based study. Clin Infect Dis 1994;19: 884–890.
6   Samore M, Magill M, Alder S, Severina E, Morrison-de Boer L, Lyon J, et al: High rates of multiple antibiotic resistance in *Streptococcus pneumoniae* from healthy children living in isolated rural communities: association with cephalosporin use and intrafamilial transmission. Pediatrics 2001;108:856–865.
7   Tan TQ, Mason EO Jr, Kaplan SL: Penicillin-resistant systemic pneumococcal infections in children: a retrospective case-control study. Pediatrics 1993;92: 761–767.
8   Lipsitch M, Levin BR: The population dynamics of antimicrobial chemotherapy. Antimicrob Agents Chemother 199741:363–373.
9   Levin BR, Lipsitch M, Perrot V, Schrag S, Antia R, Simonsen L, et al: The population genetics of antibiotic resistance. Clin Infect Dis 1997;24(suppl 1):S9–S16.
10   Harrison PF, Lederberg J (eds): Antimicrobial resistance: issues and options. Institute of Medicine workshop report. Washington, National Academy Press, 1998.
11   Barden L, Dowell S, Schwartz B, Lackey C: Current attitudes regarding use of antimicrobial agents: results from physicians' and parents' focus group discussions. Clin Pediatr 1998;37:665–671.
12   MacFarlane J, Holmes W, MacFarlane R, Britten N: Influence of patients' expectations on antibiotic management of acute lower respiratory tract illness in general practice: questionnaire study. BMJ 1997;315:1211–14.
13   Hare ME, Gaur AH, Somes GW, Arnold SR, Shorr RI: Does it really take longer not to prescribe antibiotics for viral respiratory tract infections in children? Ambul Pediatr 2006;6:152–156.
14   Coco A, Mainous AG: Relation of time spent in an encounter with the use of antibiotics in pediatric office visits for viral respiratory infections. Arch Pediatr Adolesc Med 2005;159:1145–1149.
15   Linder JA, Singer DE, Stafford RS: Association between antibiotic prescribing and visit duration in adults with upper respiratory tract infections. Clin Ther 2003;25:2419–2430.
16   Hamm RM, Hicks RJ, Bemben DA: Antibiotics and respiratory infections: are patients more satisfied when expectations are met? J Fam Pract 1996;43:56–62.
17   Gonzales R, Steiner J, Maselli J, Lum A, Barrett PH Jr: Impact of reducing antibiotic prescribing for acute bronchitis on patient satisfaction. Eff Clin Pract 2001;4:105–111.
18   Welschen I, Kuyvenhoven M, Hoes A, Verheij T: Antibiotics for acute respiratory tract symptoms: patients' expectations, GPs' management and patient satisfaction. Fam Pract 2004;21:234–237.
19   Hickner JM, Bartlett JG, Besser RE, Gonzales R, Hoffman JR, Sande MA: Principles of appropriate antibiotic use for acute rhinosinusitis in adults: background. Ann Intern Med 2001;134:498–505.
20   Arruda E, Pitkaranta A, Witek TJ Jr, Doyle CA, Hayden FG: Frequency and natural history of rhinovirus infections in adults during autumn. J Clin Microbiol 1997;35:2864–2868.
21   Finch RG, Metlay JP, Davey PG, Baker LJ: Educational interventions to improve antibiotic use in the community: report from the International Forum on Antibiotic Resistance (IFAR) colloquium, 2002. Lancet Infect Dis 2004;4:44–53.
22   Brinsley K, Sinkowitz-Cochran R, Cardo D: An assessment of issues surrounding implementation of the Campaign to Prevent Antimicrobial Resistance in Healthcare Settings. Am J Infect Control 2005;33:402–409.
23   Mainous AG, Zoorob RJ, Oler MJ, Haynes DM: Patient knowledge of upper respiratory infections: implications for antibiotic expectations and unnecessary utilization. J Fam Pract 1997;45:75–83.
24   Vanden Eng J, Marcus R, Hadler J, Imhoff B, Vugia D, Cieslak P, et al: Consumer attitudes and use of antibiotics. Emerg Infect Dis 2003;9:1128–1135.
25   Belongia EA, Naimi TS, Gale CM, Besser RE: Antibiotic use and upper respiratory infections: a survey of knowledge, attitudes, and experience in Wisconsin and Minnesota. Prev Med 2002;34:346–352.
26   Gonzales R, Wilson A, Crane LA, Barrett PH Jr: What's in a name? Public knowledge, attitudes, and experiences with antibiotic use for acute bronchitis. Am J Med 2000;108:83–85.

27 Avorn J, Solomon DH: Cultural and economic factors that (mis)shape antibiotic use: the nonpharmacologic basis of therapeutics. Ann Intern Med 2000; 133:128–135.

28 Steinman M, Gonzales R, Linder J, Landefeld C: Changing use of antibiotics in community-based outpatient practice, 1991–1999. Ann Intern Med 2003;138:525–533.

29 Mainous AG, Hueston WJ, Davis MP, Pearson WS: Trends in antimicrobial prescribing for bronchitis and upper respiratory infections among adults and children. Am J Pub Health 2003;93:1910–1914.

30 Halasa NB, Griffin MR, Zhu Y, Edwards KM: Decreased number of antibiotic prescriptions in office-based settings from 1993 to 1999 in children less than five years of age. Pediatr Infect Dis J 2002; 21:1023–1028.

31 McCaig L, Besser R, Hughes J: Trends in antimicrobial prescribing rates for children and adolescents. JAMA 2002;287:3096–3102.

32 Finkelstein JA, Stille C, Nordin J, Davis R, Raebel MA, Roblin D, et al: Reduction in antibiotic use among US children, 1996–2000. Pediatrics 2003;112: 620–627.

33 Stille CJ, Andrade SE, Huang SS, Nordin J, Raebel MA, Go AS, et al: Increased use of second-generation macrolide antibiotics for children in nine health plans in the United States. Pediatrics 2004;114:1206–1211.

34 Linder JA, Huang ES, Steinman MA, Gonzales R, Stafford RS: Fluoroquinolone prescribing in the United States: 1995 to 2002. Am J Med 2005;118:259–268.

35 Davis DA, Thomson MA, Oxman AD, Haynes RB: Changing physician performance: a systematic review of the effect of continuing medical education strategies. JAMA 1995;274:700–705.

36 Sibley JC, Sackett DL, Neufeld V, Gerrard B, Rudnick KV, Fraser W: A randomized trial of continuing medical education. N Engl J Med 1982;306:511–515.

37 Avorn J, Soumerai S: Improving drug-therapy decisions through educational outreach. N Engl J Med 1983;308:1457–1463.

38 Soumerai S, Avorn J: Principles of educational outreach ('academic detailing') to improve clinical decision making. JAMA 1990;263:549–556.

39 Arnold SR, Straus SE: Interventions to improve antibiotic prescribing practices in ambulatory care. Cochrane Database Syst Rev 2005:CD003539.

40 Gonzales R, Steiner J, Lum A, Barrett P: Decreasing antibiotic use in ambulatory practice: impact of a multidimensional intervention on the treatment of uncomplicated acute bronchitis in adults. JAMA 1999;281:1512–1518.

41 Hutchinson J, Foley R: Method of physician renumeration and rates of antibiotic prescription. CMAJ 1999;160:1013–1017.

42 Greene RA, Beckman H, Chamberlain J, Partridge G, Miller M, Burden D, et al: Increasing adherence to a community-based guideline for acute sinusitis through education, physician profiling, and financial incentives. Am J Manag Care 2004;10:670–678.

43 MacCara ME, Sketris IS, Comeau DG, Weerasinghe SD: Impact of a limited fluoroquinolone reimbursement policy on antimicrobial prescription claims. Ann Pharmacother 2001;35:852–858.

44 Belongia EA, Knobloch MJ, Kieke BA, Davis JP, Janette C, Besser RE: Impact of statewide program to promote appropriate antimicrobial drug use. Emerg Infect Dis 2005;11:912–920.

45 Schaffner W, Ray W, Federspiel C, Miller W: Improving antibiotic prescribing in office practice. JAMA 1983;250:1728–1732.

46 De Santis G, Harvey K, Howard D, Mashford M, Moulds R: Improving the quality of antibiotic prescription patterns in general practice. Med J Austral 1994;160:502–505.

47 Hux JE, Melady MP, DeBoer D: Confidential prescriber feedback and education to improve antibiotic use in primary care: a controlled trial. CMAJ 1999;161:388–392.

48 Rautakorpi UM, Huikko S, Honkanen P, Klaukka T, Makela M, Palva E, et al: The Antimicrobial Treatment Strategies (MIKSTRA) program: a 5-year follow-up of infection-specific antibiotic use in primary health care and the effect of implementation of treatment guidelines. Clin Infect Dis 2006;42: 1221–1230.

49 Samore MH, Bateman K, Alder SC, Hannah E, Donnelly S, Stoddard GJ, et al: Clinical decision support and appropriateness of antimicrobial prescribing: a randomized trial. JAMA 2005;294:2305–2314.

50 Christakis DA, Zimmerman FJ, Wright JA, Garrison MM, Rivara FP, Davis RL: A randomized controlled trial of point-of-care evidence to improve the antibiotic prescribing practices for otitis media in children. Pediatrics 2001;107:E15.

51 National Committee for Quality Assurance: The state of health care quality, 2006. Washington, NCQA, 2006.

52 Bradley NC: Expectations and experience of people who consult in a training practice. J Royal College General Practitioners 1981;31:420–425.

53 Britten N, Ukoumunne O: The influence of patients' hopes of receiving a prescription on doctors' perceptions and the decision to prescribe: a questionnaire study. BMJ 1997;315:1506–1510.

54 Cockburn J, Pit S: Prescribing behaviour in clinical practice: patients' expectations and doctors' perceptions of patients' expectations – a questionnaire study. BMJ 1997;315:520–523.

55 Himmel W, Lippert-Urbanke E, Kochen MM: Are patients more satisfied when they receive a prescription? The effect of patient expectations in general practice. Scand J Prim Health Care 1997;15:118–122.

56 Mangione-Smith R, McGlynn E, Elliott M, Krogstad P, Brook R: The relationship between perceived parental expectations and pediatrician antimicrobial prescribing behavior. Pediatrics 1999;103:711–718.

57 Stivers T, Mangione-Smith R, Elliott MN, McDonald L, Heritage J: Why do physicians think parents expect antibiotics? What parents report vs. what physicians believe. J Fam Pract 2003;52:140–148.

58 Mangione-Smith R, McGlynn EA, Elliott MN, McDonald L, Franz CE, Kravitz RL: Parent expectations for antibiotics, physician-parent communication, and satisfaction. Arch Pediatr Adolesc Med 2001;155:800–806.

59 Mangione-Smith R, Elliott MN, Stivers T, McDonald L, Heritage J, McGlynn EA: Racial/ethnic variation in parent expectations for antibiotics: implications for public health campaigns. Pediatrics 2004;113:e385–e394.

60 Scott JG, Cohen D, DiCicco-Bloom B, Orzano AJ, Jaen CR, Crabtree BF: Antibiotic use in acute respiratory infections and the ways patients pressure physicians for a prescription. J Fam Pract. 2001;50:853–858.

61 Stivers T: Presenting the problem in pediatric encounters: 'symptoms only' versus 'candidate diagnosis' presentations. Health Commun 2002;14:299–338.

62 Stivers T: Participating in decisions about treatment: overt parent pressure for antibiotic medication in pediatric encounters. Soc Sci Med 2002;54:1111–1130.

63 Stivers T: Non-antibiotic treatment recommendations: delivery formats and implications for parent resistance. Soc Sci Med 2005;60:949–964.

64 Mangione-Smith R, Elliott MN, Stivers T, McDonald L, Heritage J: Ruling out the need for antibiotics: are we sending the right message? Arch Pediatr Adolesc Med 2006;160:945–952.

65 Schwartz RK, Soumerai SB, Avorn J: Physician motivations for nonscientific drug prescribing. Soc Sci Med 1989;28:577–582.

66 Welschen I, Kuyvenhoven MM, Hoes AW, Verheij TJ: Effectiveness of a multiple intervention to reduce antibiotic prescribing for respiratory tract symptoms in primary care: randomised controlled trial. BMJ 2004;329:431.

67 Heritage J, Stivers T: Online commentary in acute medical visits: a method of shaping patient expectations. Soc Sci Med 1999;49:1501–1517.

68 Mangione-Smith R, Stivers T, Elliott M, McDonald L, Heritage J: Online commentary during the physical examination: a communication tool for avoiding inappropriate antibiotic prescribing? Soc Sci Med 2003;56:313–320.

69 Harbarth S, Albrich W, Brun-Buisson C: Outpatient antibiotic use and prevalence of antibiotic-resistant pneumococci in France and Germany: a sociocultural perspective. Emerg Infect Dis 2002;8:1460–1467.

70 Radyowijati A, Haak H: Improving antibiotic use in low-income countries: an overview of evidence on determinants. Soc Sci Med 2003;57:733–744.

71 Brixner DI: Improving acute otitis media outcomes through proper antibiotic use and adherence. Am J Manag Care 2005;11(suppl 6):S202–S210.

72 Carlson JA: Antimicrobial formulary management: meeting the challenge in a health maintenance organization. Pharmacotherapy 1991;11:32S–35S.

73 Gerbino PP, Brixner D, Sbarbaro J, Nicolau D: Appropriate antibiotic therapy for community-acquired respiratory tract infections. Manag Care Interface 2005;18:41–48.

74 MacDougall C, Polk RE: Antimicrobial stewardship programs in health care systems. Clin Microbiol Rev 2005;18:638–656.

75 Doyne EO, Alfaro MP, Siegel RM, Atherton HD, Schoettker PJ, Bernier J, et al: A randomized controlled trial to change antibiotic prescribing patterns in a community. Arch Pediatr Adolesc Med 2004;158:577–583.

76 Hennessy TW, Petersen KM, Bruden D, Parkinson AJ, Hurlburt D, Getty M, et al: Changes in antibiotic-prescribing practices and carriage of penicillin-resistant *Streptococcus pneumoniae*: a controlled intervention trial in Alaska. Clin infect Dis 2002;34:1543–1550.

77 Perz JF, Craig AS, Coffey CS, Jorgensen DM, Mitchel E, Hall S, et al: Changes in antibiotic prescribing for children after a community-wide campaign. JAMA 2002;287:3103–3109.

Edward A. Belongia, MD
Epidemiology Research Center (ML2)
Marshfield Clinic Research Foundation
1000 North Oak Avenue, Marshfield, WI 54449 (USA)
Tel. +1 715 389 3783, Fax +1 715 389 3880, E-Mail belongia.edward@marshfieldclinic.org

Weber JT (ed): Antimicrobial Resistance – Beyond the Breakpoint.
Issues Infect Dis. Basel, Karger, 2010, vol 6, pp 89–101

# Reducing Antimicrobial-Resistant Infections in Health Care Settings: What Works?

Katayoun Rezai · Robert A. Weinstein

John H. Stroger Hospital, Division of Infectious Diseases, Chicago Ill., USA

## Abstract

Antimicrobial resistance is a major public health concern worldwide, especially in health care facilities. Resistance is driven by inadequate hospital hygiene (especially lapses in hand washing), selective pressures due to over-usage of antibiotics, failures of host immunity and mobile genetic elements that can encode bacterial resistance. Alcohol-based hand rubs are effective and time saving for health care workers and offer the chance to greatly improve hand hygiene adherence. Antibiotic stewardship and computer-based ordering are the most effective interventions to improve antibiotic use. Identification and isolation of the 'resistance iceberg' is often used, especially for outbreak control. Cleansing patients and disinfecting the environment can contribute to control efforts. Prevention of device-related infections may provide the best return on investment for control of resistance. A number of novel approaches to resistance control are on the horizon; however, basic infection control tenets offer the best approach for the present.



## Overview

Antimicrobial resistance in health care facilities is a global public health concern. Over 70% of bacterial pathogens found in US hospitals are resistant to at least 1 antibiotic, and more than 14,000 patients die annually from resistant nosocomial infections. Antimicrobial-resistant microorganisms can be associated with increased mortality and morbidity, prolonged hospital stay and higher costs. For example, patients with bacteremia caused by methicillin-resistant *Staphylococcus aureus* (MRSA) have longer hospitalizations and higher hospital costs and mortality than do patients with bacteremia caused by methicillin-susceptible *S. aureus*. Fear of resistance leads physicians to prescribe newer, more expensive antibiotics, costing at least USD 4–5 billion in 1998 in the United States. The combination of highly susceptible patients, prolonged and complex antibiotic use, cross infection due to poor infection control practices (especially lapses in hand hygiene), and shuttling of patients infected with resistant pathogens between nursing homes and hospitals has resulted in nosocomial infections with highly resistant strains.

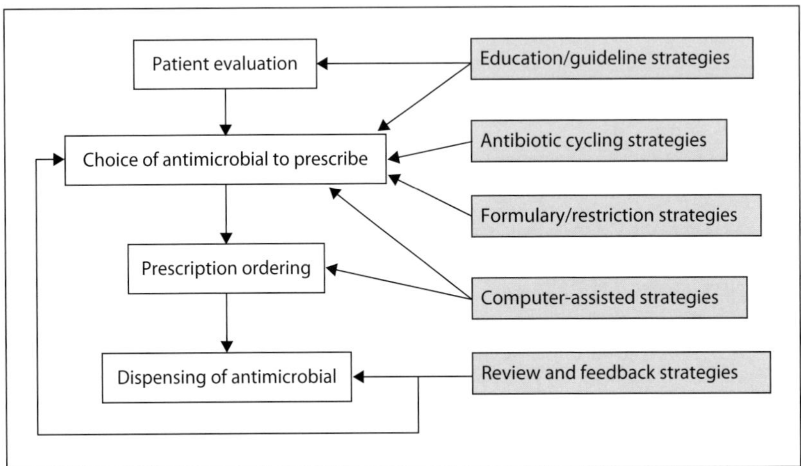


**Fig. 1.** Antimicrobial prescribing process and antimicrobial stewardship strategies. From MacDougall and Polk [1].

The goals of this chapter are to review factors that contribute to nosocomial antimicrobial resistance and to outline approaches to control, prevention and eradication of antimicrobial resistance in health care settings.

## Antibiotic Control

### Starting Antibiotics

Many of the factors related to antimicrobial resistance stem from the misuse of antimicrobials. Twenty-five million pounds of antibiotics are produced each year, and these drugs are administered to 30–50% of hospitalized patients. Surveys have shown that as much as 50% of all antimicrobial use is inappropriate.

Improving antimicrobial use can be defined as ensuring the optimal selection, dosage and duration of antimicrobial treatment that results in the best clinical outcome for the treatment and prevention of infection, with minimal toxicity to the patient and minimal impact on subsequent resistance [1] (fig. 1). This goal could be achieved when an infectious process is identified accurately with appropriate culture and susceptibility testing; then the appropriate treatment modalities are applied which include the right antibiotic, removal of unneeded or infected invasive devices, and debridement and drainage of infected tissue. The initial choice of antibiotic should be based on the knowledge of hospital- and ward-specific antimicrobial susceptibility patterns.

Many strategies have been developed to manage institutional antibiotic use, based on observations that lessening antibiotic pressures can lead to improvements in resistance patterns. The milestone study by Price and Sleigh [2] showed that complete cessation of antibiotic usage on a neurosurgical intensive care unit (ICU) ended an outbreak of multidrug-resistant *Klebsiella* infection and reduced the rate of infection with other organisms. Most intervention studies aimed at control of resistant organisms also have included improved infection control efforts and have had quasi-experimental 'before/after' study designs, making it difficult to attribute cause and effect entirely to the antibiotic controls. Often, the 2 measures, antibiotic and infection control, are interrelated and difficult to separate, both in practice and in analysis of impact.

In one study, a restrictive antibiotic policy was introduced in response to a nosocomial outbreak of multi-resistant *Acinetobacter* spp. that persisted despite infection-control procedures. Prior approval was required for use of amikacin, ceftazidime, ciprofloxacin, fluconazole, oflaxacin or ticarcillin/clavulanate, even in ICUs. Resistant *Acinetobacter* and also many β-lactam- or fluroquinolone-resistant Enterobacteriaceae were controlled, and there was a 32% decrease in expenditure for parenteral antibiotics. Researchers noted no detrimental effect on survival, time to discharge, length of ICU stay or time to receive appropriate antibiotics despite the restrictions. The cost of implementing the policy was less than USD 150,000 per year and the projected annual savings were USD 900,000 [3]. Using less restrictive policies (i.e. real-time review of orders and feedback to prescribers by a pharmacist and/or infectious diseases fellow), one group noted 50% of patients initially treated with costly parenteral antibiotics had their regimens refined and that the modifications resulted in significant reductions in antibiotic expenses without sacrificing patient care [4].

The era of electronic information technology has made computer provider order entry an option for effecting antibiotic stewardship. Computer programs offer the medical provider guidance in a non-judgmental and fact-based format and can change the prescribing habits of the clinicians dramatically. Evans et al. [5] devised a computer-assisted program, linked to patients' electronic medical records, that provides detailed recommendations and warnings to prescribing clinicians. In a 12 month study of that system, there was a significant reduction in prescribed antibiotic doses, side effects, costs and durations of hospital stay [5].


*Duration of Antibiotic Therapy*


Even with optimal antibiotic choices, duration of therapy may drive resistance. ICUs are resistance epicenters. About 62% of patients in the ICU receive antimicrobials; half receive more than one antibiotic, and ~65% are treated for pulmonary infections, which are present in only 35–75% of those being treated. In one study, in order to minimize the excessive use of antimicrobials in treatment of ventilator-associated pneumonia (VAP), a predictive clinical pulmonary infection score (CPIS) – a simple score based on temperature, white blood cell count, character of pulmonary secretions, $O_2$ requirements, and diffuseness of infiltrates – was devised. Patients with a CPIS <6 were treated with ciprofloxacin monotherapy for 72 h and if the score remained <6, ciprofloxacin was discontinued. Eighty percent of those patients with low scores when therapy was started maintained low scores (i.e. putative absence of VAP), were able to stop antibiotics, and did well [6]. Further studies are required to validate the use of the CPIS and efficacy of shorter duration of antibiotics in VAP. Of note, in a multi-center trial, patients with VAP were randomized to 8 versus 15 days of antibiotic therapy [7]. The primary outcome measures – death from any cause, micro-biologically documented pulmonary infection recurrence and antibiotic-free days – were assessed 28 days after VAP onset. The outcomes were similar for both groups. However, among those patients with recurrent infection, multi-resistant pathogens emerged less frequently in patients treated for 8 versus15 days (42.1 vs. 62%) [7].

*Antibiotic Rotation*

Antibiotic rotation is an old intervention that has re-emerged in an attempt to con-trol resistance, particularly in closed units such as ICUs. Antibiotic cycling is based on deliberate removal and substitution of antimicrobial classes to avoid monolithic selective pressures and hopefully decrease or reverse the emergence of resistance. The hypothesis is that if resistance occurs to one antibiotic over a period of time, expo-sure to another antibiotic with different mechanism of action and resistance for the next period will remove any advantage for the resistant organisms. The potential for application of this theory was illustrated by Gerding [8], who due to high rates of gen-tamicin resistance among Gram-negative bacilli, substituted amikacin for gentamicin in the hospital formulary at 2 separate points in a 10-year period at the Minneapolis Veterans Affairs Medical Center. Coincident with these formulary changes, there were significant decreases in the rate of gentamicin resistance in Gram-negative bacilli [8].

Martinez et al. [9] compared monthly cycling to patient-level mixing strategies in 2 ICUs. Cefepime-resistant *Pseudomonas aeruginosa* occurred more frequently dur-ing mixing (9%) versus cycling (3%), but methodologic issues may have lessened the validity of this finding and of the results of the other cycling studies. Most cycling studies have had limited effect on overall antibiotic use and adherence to cycling usually has been incomplete. The jury remains out on the value of this strategy.

## Infection-Control Practices

*Hand Hygiene*

Nosocomial transmission of pathogens, including resistant organisms, is attributed in large part to poor hand hygiene by personnel (compliance level), number of con-tacts (contact rate) and high 'colonization pressure' (frequency of bacterial carriage by adjacent patients). Hand hygiene is cited as the single most important nosocomial infection control measure; however, adherence is very low, often not more than 25–50%. The major features associated with poor adherence have been inadequate time due to heavy workloads, intensity of care, time of day, low nurse-to-patient ratios and avoidance of adverse skin effects caused by repeated hand washing.

Efforts to insure adherence mostly have used educational programs, hand hygiene campaigns, and a focus on use of emollient-rich alcohol-based hand rub rather than soap-and-water (to decrease deleterious effects on skin). Effective hand washing with soap and water requires 45–90 s and a sink. Alcohol-based hand rubs take 10–30 s, can be applied as health care workers move between patients and do not require a sink. In order to generate high compliance, programs may benefit from a combination of educational campaigns, observation and direct health care worker feedback, development of a sense of personal responsibility by health care workers, and sanctions for non-adherence. Although, at least in the short run, use of alcohol hand rub has not resolved the issue of adherence, persistence and insistence by hospital leaders, including enforced remedial infection control education for health care workers who are not adherent, may improve hand hygiene rates.

Universal gloving has been shown to decrease the chance of health care worker hand contamination with patients' flora by 70–80%, and it can be an important adjunct to hand hygiene to control transmission of resistant organisms. As colonization pressure increases, very high hand hygiene adherence will be needed to control cross-transmission. In the landmark study of the role of colonization pressure in the spread of vancomycin-resistant *Enterococcus* (VRE), time to acquisition of VRE was shorter with high colonization pressure [10]. In such settings, universal gloving may be particularly valuable.

*Gowns*

Health care workers hands may not be the only source of transmission. The contaminated clothing of health care workers may also contribute to transmission of organisms. One study showed that 37% of health care worker's gowns were contaminated with VRE after care of a colonized patient. Another study has shown that 40% of the time, health care workers' gowns were contaminated with MRSA or VRE after caring for colonized patients and that gowns prevented clothing contamination. 'White coats' become contaminated with VRE or MRSA after examining a patient and the organisms may be transferred to the health care workers' hands 27% of the time after touching the coat [11]. In some health care settings, long-sleeved clothing has been banned for infection control purposes.

Boyce et al. [12] showed containment of an outbreak of VRE only after mandating that health care workers wear gowns when caring for patients with VRE. However, that study described a clonal (single-strain) outbreak, used historical controls, and did not monitor compliance with glove or gown precautions at baseline or during the intervention periods [12]. Several studies have shown lower rates of patients becoming culture-positive when health care workers wore gowns and gloves compared to gloves only. At least one of the studies had implemented multiple interventions, including decreased use of cephalosporin and clindamycin in addition to gowning, so it is difficult to attribute the decreased rate solely to gowning. Slaughter et al. [13] in a trial that was methodologically more rigorous, showed universal gloving to be as effective as use of gowns and gloves for control of endemic VRE. Gowning may be most useful in hospitals where there is a single-strain outbreak or when environmental contamination is high [13].

*Source Control*

*Patient Cleansing*

Decontamination of patients' skin and the environment also can be important infection-control measures. VRE can be transferred from contaminated sites in the environment or on patients' intact skin to clean sites via health care worker hands or gloves in 11% of opportunities. An adjunctive approach to reducing risks of cross-transmission is 'source control' by decontamination of patients' skin. In the 1970s, a retrospective study in response to a US Food and Drug Administration requirement to discontinue cleansing neonates with hexachlorophene suggested that such cleansing had prevented outbreaks of neonatal staphylococcal disease. Using antiseptics, such as octonedine dihydrochloride, chlorhexidine or triclosan, for whole-body washing, investigators have demonstrated a reduction in rates of colonization and infection with MRSA in hospitalized patients.

In 2 recent studies, 2% chlorhexidine gluconate was used to cleanse patients in medical ICUs. Compared to soap-and-water bathing, chlorhexidine cleanings reduced levels of VRE on patients' skin, on health care workers' hands, and on environmental surfaces. Rates of bloodstream infections also were markedly reduced [14]. Potential problems – development of chlorhexidine-resistant organisms or occurrence of allergic reactions – were not observed in these studies [14]. Source control, for example with chlorhexidine, can be an important adjunctive measure to reduce transmission of and infections due to resistant organisms in ICUs.

*Environmental Disinfection*

Hospitalized patients are surrounded by devices, equipment and environmental surfaces from which antimicrobial-resistant organisms can be recovered frequently. Equipment carried by health care workers (e.g. stethoscopes, tourniquets, otoscopes and pagers) can become contaminated and may act as potential vectors for transmission of resistant organisms. Environmental contamination is a particular problem when microbes have environmental durability. VRE, *Acinetobacter*, and *Clostridium difficile* can persist on hospital surfaces and equipement – bed rails, ear and rectal probe thermometers, pulse oximeters, doorknobs, tables over beds, wheelchairs, linens and computer keyboards – for days to months.

*S. aureus* also has been isolated from a variety of equipment and environmental surfaces, stethoscopes, tables over beds, blood pressure cuffs, hydrotherapy tanks, mops and charts. One study found that 73% of the hospital rooms containing patients infected with MRSA (and 69% containing colonized patients) had environmental contamination with MRSA [15]. The gloves of the nurses were contaminated with MRSA 42% of the time just by touching a room surface [15]. In burn units, exposure to contaminated surfaces or therapy tanks has been identified as a risk factor for transmission of resistant bacteria.

The environment as the source of transmission of infection has not been the focus of many intervention studies. Hayden et al. [16] used VRE as a marker organism, investigating the effects of improved environmental cleaning with and without promotion of hand hygiene adherence on the spread of VRE in a medical ICU. The investigators concluded that improving environmental cleaning from 48–87% of monitored sites cleaned led to a reduction in the rate of VRE acquisition of >60%.

Decreasing environmental contamination can help to control the spread of VRE and possibly other resistant pathogens in hospitals. When developing cleaning policies, health care facilities should consider the amount of contact with patients, for example areas with frequent hand contact such as bed rails and door knobs may be targeted for cleaning and monitoring [17].

*Disinfectants*

Most surface disinfectants, such as quaternary ammonium compounds and phenolics, are active against resistant organisms such as MRSA and VRE; however, the disinfectants need to be used in proper amounts and dilutions, and contact times with surfaces need to be sufficient and consistent [17]. Some equipment and instruments – such as stethoscopes, blood pressure cuffs and other portable equipment – could be cleaned with 70% isopropyl alcohol, which decreases the bacterial counts significantly [17].

Silver and its compounds have been used as antimicrobial agents since the 1800s. Silver sulfadiazine is the most common form of silver compound used for burns. Silver-based compounds also have been studied for environmental disinfection. Brady et al. [18] compared the durability and efficacy of silver disinfectant to more common disinfectants, such as quaternary ammonium disinfectants. Silver disinfectant had the greatest antimicrobial kinetics and spectrum of activity with a persistent antimicrobial residue.

Silver is also being studied as an antimicrobial powder which could be applied on surfaces. This technology has been used in Japan in ceramics containing silver ions in the form of silver zeolite and silver zirconium phosphate for food preservation, disinfection of medical supplies, and decontamination of surfaces of medical equipment, kitchenware and toys. The silver and zinc-containing matrix (AgION) as a coating for stainless steel was tested for antimicrobial efficacy against *Escherichia coli, S. aureus, Pseudomonas* and *Listeria monocytogenes.* AgION reduced microbial colony-forming units when compared to uncoated steel surfaces under all conditions; furthermore, powder-coated surfaces retained a high degree of activity after 5 cycles of cleaning with soap and water or dry towel dusting. Silver as a disinfectant coating for hospital and clinic environmental surfaces such as door knobs, bed rails, counters and instruments warrants evaluation to assess its efficacy and durability.

*Potable Water*
Waterborne nosocomial outbreaks have been described in multiple studies. Reuter et al. [19] showed that in their ICU, 35% of all cases of acquired colonization with *P. aeruginosa* originated from contaminated tap water and that retrograde contamination of faucets by patients occurred in 15% of cases. They conclude that contamination of faucets with *P. aeruginosa* is an important source of endemic *P. aeruginosa* [19]. Use of alcohol-based hand rubs rather than soap and water for routine hand disinfection by all health care workers may reduce transmission from faucets.

**Isolation Precautions**

Attempts to control the spread of resistant organisms rely on improving use of antibiotics, increasing hand hygiene among health care workers and identifying and isolating patients who harbor resistant organisms. Such patients are not always infected or symptomatic; the majority may just be colonized. Identification of the silent reservoir of resistant organism (the 'resistance iceberg') could be accomplished by active surveillance and implementation of contact precaution, which can help to prevent the spread of resistance (fig. 2) [20].

Many studies have shown that in the setting of multiple (simultaneous or sequential) interventions, implementation of surveillance cultures to identify colonized patients has led to a significant reduction in rates of colonization and infection of patients with MRSA or VRE. One study compared the rate of transmission of MRSA from colonized patients who were identified by active surveillance and placed in contact precaution with that from patients who were colonized but not yet identified or isolated. The rate of transmission was 15.6-fold higher for patients not identified to be colonized and for whom standard precautions were being used [21].

*Active Surveillance and Isolation*

In order for isolation measures to work, the resistant organism must be recognized. The importance of active surveillance for colonization and not relying on routine

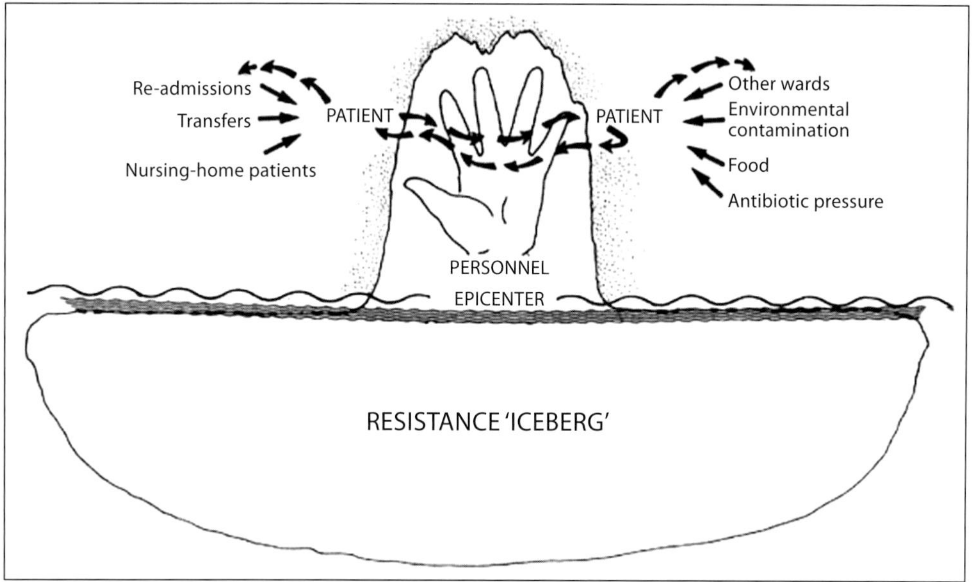

**Fig. 2.** Dynamics of nosocomial resistance. Many resistant bacteria colonize patients in an occult manner and are spread from patient to patient on hands of health care workers. The other factors (e.g. environmental contamination) contribute to the spread of resistant bacteria. Adapted from Weinstein and Kabins [20].

microbiological cultures from infections has been demonstrated in a hospital with an MRSA outbreak. A clonal outbreak of MRSA in a hospital was the cause of 40% of all hospital-acquired *S. aureus* bloodstream infections and 49% of all *S. aureus* surgical-site infections. During the first 3 years of the outbreak, patients with MRSA were identified for isolation mainly by diagnostic cultures. The incidence of infection and prevalence of colonization with MRSA continued to rise. Once active surveillance cultures were implemented to detect and isolate patients colonized but not yet infected by the outbreak strain, the rate of colonization and infection dropped significantly [22].

The relative contribution of active surveillance cultures and isolation to control of resistance has been debated. The Society for Healthcare Epidemiology of America (SHEA) recommended routine use of active surveillance cultures and contact precautions for control of VRE and MRSA; however, the Centers for Disease Control and Prevention (CDC) isolation guidelines recommend this as one of several approaches to be implemented based on evaluation of impact of control efforts [17]. A review of studies on effectiveness of active surveillance and isolation measures in management of MRSA in hospitals described major methodological weaknesses. In most studies, multiple interventions were introduced at the same time, therefore the role of active surveillance and isolation measures alone could not be assessed [23]. Moreover, several studies have shown that patients placed in isolation were seen about half as often as patients who were not in isolation, which particularly means less frequent care and possibly a psychological sense of isolation and which may suggest the mechanism by which active surveillance cultures and isolation contain MRSA (i.e. no contact, no transmission).

*Rapid Detection*

Although the jury may be out on effectiveness of active surveillance and isolation in controlling endemic resistant-organism spread, studies have shown that in outbreak settings these measures along with other interventions are important to control the outbreak. Technology may aid in efforts to control spread of resistant bacteria. Rapid and sensitive DNA-based tests for detection of resistant organisms such as MRSA and VRE may facilitate the identification of patients who are colonized or infected. But the infection control cost-benefit of such molecular probes has not been demonstrated.

In addition, availability of electronic medical records could make the process of identification ('flagging'), notification and tracking of the carriers of resistant organisms more efficient, convenient and accurate, so that appropriate infection control measures can be implemented.

## Prevention of Infection to Prevent Resistance

*Device-Related Infections*

The application of infection control measures to prevent spread of resistant organisms may never be perfect, and even when control of resistance is nearly perfect there has been a striking lack of correlation of resistance and overall nosocomial infection rates. For example, those countries which have used active surveillance to almost eliminate MRSA have overall nosocomial infection rates similar to those of the United States, where MRSA is often rampant. This suggests that greater emphasis should be placed on prevention of infection, specifically related to devices.

Prevention of central venous catheter (CVC)-related infection has been under extensive study. In the United States, approximately 80,000 CVC-related bloodstream infections, representing 5.3 infections per 1,000 catheter days, are reported annually in ICUs [24]. Mortality associated with these infections ranges from 10–25%. CDC guidelines for prevention of CVC-related bloodstream infections based on evidence-based research emphasize 5 preventive measures: educating personnel about inserting lines; removing catheters that are not needed or not used; chlorhexidine prep for disinfection of the site; using maximum barrier precautions during catheter insertion; and use of antiseptic- or anti-infective-coated catheters if after full implementation of all the above, the goals are not met [24]. 'Bundling' such interventions, each of which is evidence-based, can virtually eliminate CVC-related bloodstream infections, even without use of anti-infective catheters. The future of preventing device related infections may be in recent advances made in understanding bacterial pathogenicity and identification of virulence factors. Bacteria communicate with each other through specific signaling chemicals to act as a community, rather than individual cells, to achieve a critical density or a 'quorum'. Once the quorum has been established, it can signal to turn on a variety of virulence factors that are essential for dissemination of the organisms and to form biofilms, that are considered to be integral to development of catheter-related infections. Prevention of quorum-sensing to prevent biofilm formation may be the future of prevention of catheter-related infections.

*Host Defense*

Prevention of infection also depends on the host defense system. Making the host less susceptible to infection could prevent infection. One very productive area of research has been on tight glucose control and prevention of infection post-operatively or in ICUs. Continuous i.v. insulin infusion produced a significant decrease in the risk of deep sternal wound infection after coronary artery bypass surgery. Intensive glucose control with i.v. insulin has also been shown in a randomized control trial to significantly reduce sepsis and other morbidities in critically ill patients [25], though this has not been a universal finding.

**Future Approaches**

Future approaches may focus on systems, cells and vaccines. First, it is conventional wisdom that bioinformatics will facilitate and reduce the time to retrieve appropriate and needed information, can be harnessed to provide patient-specific recommendations that will help physicians make sound decisions, and will assist monitoring patients with resistant organisms. This conventional wisdom now needs to be widely applied and tested.

Second, a cellular approach to combat resistance may be to 'cure resistant bacteria' through genetic modification. For example, when plasmids that contain synthetic genes coding for small oligoribonucleotides (called external guide sequences or EGSs) are introduced into antibiotic-resistant *E. coli*, the EGSs complex with mRNA encoded by genes responsible for drug resistance; when the complexes are cleaved, resistance is inactivated [26].

Third, development of vaccines against nosocomial bacteria for high-risk patients is the Holy Grail quest. A conjugate vaccine conferred partial immunity against *S. aureus* bacteremia in hemodialysis patients for 40 days but durable immunity was not achieved.

Of value in endemic settings
- Appropriate antibiotic selection and antibiotic restriction
- Shortening duration of antibiotic courses when possible
- Hand hygiene with alcohol-based hand rub
- Universal gloving
- Patient cleansing with chlorhexidine gluconate in medical intensive care units
- Environmental decontamination
- Prevention of device-related infection using HICPAC/CDC guidelines
- Augmenting host defense when feasible (e.g. improved glucose control)

Of added value in epidemics and some endemic settings
- Gowns for contact isolation
- Active surveillance cultures to direct contact precautions for the 'resistance iceberg'

Jury is out – *caveat emptor*
- Antibiotic rotation

Promising – need further evaluation
- Decolonization of colonized patients or health care workers
- Silver disinfectant coating (e.g. catheter, environmental surfaces)
- 'Curing bacterial resistance' via genetic modification
- Vaccines against nosocomial organism
- Prevention of quorum-sensing to prevent biofilm formation

Despite these prospects for a bold new future, it is unlikely that avant garde interventions will eliminate resistant organisms completely. We need to continue to promote and ensure adherence to the basic and essential principles of infection control and asepsis discussed in this chapter (table 1).

## References

1 MacDougall C, Polk RE: Antimicrobial stewardship programs in health care systems. Clin Microbiol Rev 2005;18:638–656.

2 Price DJ, Sleigh JD: Control of infection due to *Klebsiella aerogenes* in neurosurgical unit by withdrawarl of all anitbioitcs. Lancet 1970;2:1213–1215.

3 White AC Jr., Atmar RL, Wilson J, et al: Effects of requiring prior authorization for selected antimicrobials; expenditure, susceptibilities and clinical outcomes. Clin Infect Dis 1997;25:230–239.

4 Fraser GL, Stogsdill P, Dickens JD Jr, et al: Antibiotic optimization: an evaluation of patient safety and economic outcomes. Arch Intern Med 1997;157: 1689–1694.

5 Evans RS, Pestotnik SL, Classen DC, et al: A computer-assisted management program for antibiotics and other antiinfective agents. N Engl J Med 1998; 338:232–238.

6 Singh N, Rogers P, Atwood CW, et al: Short-course empiric antibiotic therapy for patients with pulmonary infiltrates in the intensive care unit: a proposed solution for indiscriminate antibiotic prescription. Am J Respir Crit Care Med 2000;162:505–511.

7 Chastre J Wolff M, Fagon JY, et al: Comparison of 8 vs 15 days of antibiotic therapy for ventilator-associated pneumonia in adults: a randomized trial. JAMA 2003;290:2588–2598.

8   Gerding DN; Antimicrobial cycling: lessons learned from the aminoglycoside experience. Infect Control Hosp Epidemiol 2000;21(suppl 1):S12–S17.

9   Martinez JA, Nicolas JM, Marco F, et al: Comparison of antimicrobial cycling and mixing strategies in two medical intensive care units. Crit Care Med 2006; 34:329–336.

10  Bonten MJ, Slaughter S, Ambergen AW, et al: The role of 'colonization pressure' in the spread of vancomycin-resistant enterococci: an important infection control variable. Arch Intern Med 1998;158: 1127–1132.

11  Boyce JM, Chenevert C: Isolation gowns prevent health care workers from contaminating their clothing, and possibly their hands, with methicillin-resistant *Staphylococcus aureus* (MRSA) and resistant enterococci. Eighth Ann Meet Soc Healthcare Epidemiol Am, 1998.

12  Boyce JM, Opal SM, Chow JW, et al: Outbreak of multidrug-resistant *Enterococcus faecium* with transferable vanB class vancomycin resistance. J Clin Microbiol 1994;32:1148–1153.

13  Slaughter S, Hayden MK, Nathan C, et al: A comparison of the effect of universal use of gloves and gowns with that of glove use alone on acquisition of vancomycin-resistant enterococci in a medical intensive care unit. Ann Int Med 1996;125:448–456.

14  Bleasdale SC, Trick WE, Gonzalez IM, et al: Effectiveness of chlorhexidine bathing to reduce catheter-associated bloodstream infections in medical intensive care unit patients. Arch Intern Med 2007;167:2073–2079.

15  Boyce JM, Potter-Bynoe G, Chenevert C, et al: Environmental contamination due to methicillin-resistant *Staphylococcus aureus*: possible infection control implications. Infect Control Hosp Epidemiol 1997;18:622–627.

16  Hayden MK, Bonten MJ, Blom DW, et al: Reduction in acquisition of vancomycin-resistant *Enterococcus* after enforcement of routine environmental cleaning measures. Clin Infect Dis 2006;42:1552–1560.

17  Muto CA, Jernigan JA, Ostrowsky BE, et al: SHEA guideline for preventing nosocomial transmission of multidrug-resistant strains of *Staphylococcus aureus* and *Enterococcus*. Infect Control Hosp Epidemiol 2003;24:362–386.

18  Brady MJM, Lisay CM, et al: Persistent silver disinfectant for the environmental control of pathogenic bacteria. Am J Infect Control 2003;31:208–214.

19  Reuter S, Sigge A, Wiedeck H, et al: Analysis of transmission pathways of *Pseudomonas aeruginosa* between patients and tap water outlets. Crit Care Med 2002;30:2222–2228.

20  Weinstein RA, Kabins SA: Strategies for prevention and control of multiple drug-resistant nosocomial infection. Am J Med 1981;70:449–454.

21  Jernigan JA, Titus MG, Gröschel DH, et al: Effectiveness of contact isolation during a hospital outbreak of methicillin-resistant *Staphylococcus aureus*. Am J Epidemiol 1996;143:496–504.

22  Thompson RL, Cabezudo I, Wenzel RP: Epidemiology of nosocomial infections caused by methicillin-resistant *Staphylococcus aureus*. Ann Intern Med 1982; 97:309–317.

23  Cooper BS, Stone SP, Kibbler CC, et al: Isolation measures in the hospital management of methicillin resistant *Staphylococcus aureus* (MRSA): systematic review of the literature. BMJ 2004;329:533.

24  O'Grady NP, et al: Guidelines for the Prevention of Intravascular Catheter–Related Infections. Guidelines 2002;35:1281.

25  Van den Berghe G, Wouters P, Weekers F, et al: Intensive insulin therapy in critically ill patients. N Engl J Med 2001;345:1359–1367.

26  Cecilia Guerrier-Takada RS, Altman S: Phenotypic conversion of drug-resistant bacteria to drug sensitivity. Proc Natl Acad Sci USA 1997;94:8468–8472.

Katayoun Rezai, MD
John H. Stroger Hospital
Division of Infectious Diseases
637 South Wood Street, Chicago IL 60612 (USA)
Tel. +1 312 864 4552, Fax +1 312 864 9496, E-Mail krezai@rush.edu

Weber JT (ed): Antimicrobial Resistance – Beyond the Breakpoint.
Issues Infect Dis. Basel, Karger, 2010, vol 6, pp 102–119

# Cost of Antimicrobial Resistance in Healthcare Settings: A Critical Review

Liana R. Merz[a] · Rebecca M. Guth[a] · Victoria J. Fraser[a,b]

[a]Division of Infectious Diseases, Washington University School of Medicine, and [b]Barnes Jewish Hospital, St. Louis, Mo., USA

## Abstract

Antibiotic resistant bacteria are a significant problem of public health importance, and are responsible for substantial hospital morbidity, mortality and cost. Estimates of cost vary, however, depending on the organism of interest, the study design and other factors. Most previous cost studies focused on antibiotic resistance as it impacts healthcare facility costs. Differences in design and methods make comparisons between these studies difficult, and there are clear limitations in the methodology frequently used in these analyses. Significant improvement is needed in studies of the cost of antimicrobial resistance, including more rigorous design and analytical methods, to generate more reliable estimates of the real cost of antibiotic resistance. Collaboration with economic experts will aid in producing more accurate cost estimates that can be used to guide healthcare administration decisions and resource utilization.



Antibiotic-resistant bacteria are an increasing problem of public health importance in both hospital and community settings. According to the Centers for Disease Control and Prevention's (CDC) National Healthcare Safety Network (NHSN) in 2007, 56.2% of *S. aureus* isolates were resistant to oxacillin and 33.3% of enterococci were resistant to vancomycin [1]. Begun in 2005 and replacing the National Nosocomial Infections Surveillance System (NNIS), the NHSN is a voluntary national surveillance system that tracks patient and healthcare personnel safety. The NHSN data demonstrate that antibiotic resistance continues to increase significantly in hospitals and especially in intensive care units (ICUs). When comparing NNIS antibiotic susceptibility data from 1998–2002 to data from 2003, there was a 12% increase in enterococci resistance to vancomycin and an 11% increase in *S. aureus* resistance to methicillin. Resistance in *Klebsiella pneumoniae* and *Pseudomonas aeruginosa* to third generation cephalosporins increased 47 and 20%, respectively, during the same time frame [2].

According to the CDC, 70% of bacteria causing hospital-acquired infections are resistant to at least one of the antibiotics commonly used to treat healthcare associated infections [3]. Previous studies have shown antibiotic-resistant infections to be associated with increased length of hospital stay and cost, and increased attributable mortality, although results vary [4–9]. Methods, designs and outcomes of studies on antibiotic-resistant organisms vary among the published literature. Despite the increasing prevalence of antibiotic-resistant organisms, their full health and economic impacts have not been adequately explored [7]. There is a need to perform more extensive research on the economic impact and outcomes of antibiotic resistance in diverse settings.

## Global Estimates of Cost

Questions are often raised about what should be considered a part of the cost of antimicrobial resistance. In the United States, the Office of Technology Assessment estimated that the incremental cost of antimicrobial resistance in hospitals was USD 661 million (in 1992 dollars), but this estimate only included the marginal costs associated with antibiotic-resistant infections. If all costs, including fixed costs and the increased drug costs associated with changing empiric therapy were included, this estimate would have been larger. Current estimates place the national costs of antimicrobial resistance between USD 100 million and USD 30 billion annually in the United States [10].

## Perspective

Previous research on antimicrobial resistance has considered cost from the perspective of the hospital and health-care system, since these costs are more readily available for analysis. Direct costs of resistance include spending on isolating patients, staffing (nurses, doctors, infection control practitioners, etc.), laboratory tests, antimicrobials and patient procedures, as well as the additional expense associated with increased length of hospital stay [11]. While this approach is valuable, it may also be important to include impacts outside of the hospital, including time spent in nursing homes, lost wages and other indirect costs. Society ultimately pays the price for increased resistance, in terms of disease burden and quality of life, but hospitals in particular are responsible for funding interventions to stem the spread of resistant organisms.

## Literature Review

*Methicillin-Resistant Staphylococcus aureus*

In terms of cost, MRSA is by far the most studied antibiotic-resistant organism (table 1). Reported costs vary widely between studies due to differences in study populations,

**Table 1.** The economic cost associated with methicillin-resistant *Staphylococcus aureus*

| Year | First author [Ref] | Population | Sample size, n | Type of infection | Cost results |
|---|---|---|---|---|---|
| 1988 | Wakefield [12] | tertiary-care, teaching hospital inpatients | 58 | multiple | mean cost of MRSA infection (USD 7,481) significantly higher than MSSA (USD 2,377, p < 0.001) |
| 1999 | Abramson [18] | tertiary-care, teaching hospital inpatients | 38 | bloodstream | attributable cost of MRSA bloodstream infection (USD 27,083) significantly higher than MSSA bloodstream infection (USD 9,661, p = 0.043) |
| 1999 | Chaix [19] | urban tertiary-care teaching hospital: medical ICU patients | 54 | multiple | mean attributable cost of MRSA infection was USD 9,725 compared to patients without MRSA colonization or infection |
| 1999 | Rubin [13] | administrative data: inpatients from New York City hospitals | 13,550 | multiple | cost difference between MRSA and MSSA patients was USD 2,500 |
| 2001 | Kim [45] | urban tertiary-care teaching hospital inpatients | 20 | multiple | attributable cost to treat a MRSA infection was USD 14,360 |
| 2003 | Capitano [16] | long-term care facility residents | 90 | multiple | infection cost for MRSA (USD 2,607) higher than infection cost for MSSA (USD 1,332, p<0.001) |
| 2003 | Engemann [9] | tertiary-care teaching hospital surgical inpatients | 479 | surgical site infection | MRSA SSI associated with additional cost of USD 13,901 compared to MSSA SSI |
| 2004 | Kopp [21] | inpatients | 72 | multiple | median hospital cost of patients with MSSA (USD 12,862) less than that of MRSA patients (USD 16,575), but not significant (p = 0.11) |
| 2004 | McHugh [4] | urban tertiary-care hospital inpatients | 60 | bloodstream | USD 5,302 higher cost per patient day for MRSA patients compared to MSSA patients for patients with a Case Mix Index >2 |
| 2005 | Cosgrove [22] | urban teaching hospital inpatients | 348 | bloodstream | USD 3,836 average attributable hospital cost for patients with MRSA |

| Year | First author [Ref] | Population | Sample size, n | Type of infection | Cost results |
|---|---|---|---|---|---|
| 2005 | Lodise [24] | urban teaching hospital inpatients | 273 | bloodstream | cost of MRSA infection (USD 21,577) significantly higher than MSSA infection (USD 11,668, p = 0.001) |
| 2005 | Reed [23] | teaching hospital hemodialysis inpatients | 143 | bloodstream | mean adjusted costs for MRSA (USD 21,251) significantly higher than MSSA (USD 13,978, p=0.012) |
| 2009 | Ben-David [25] | tertiary care hospital inpatients | 182 consecutive patients | bloodstream | significant difference found using multivariate analysis (higher cost following infection: USD 17,603 vs. USD 51,492); difference not significant when using propensity scoring |

sample sizes and methods, which makes direct comparisons of these studies difficult. However, there are clear limitations to many of the studies currently available.

Early studies of costs attributable to MRSA were relatively unsophisticated in their design and analyses, but they do shed light on an increasing concern. Wakefield et al. [12] examined 58 patients with *S. aureus* infection at a university hospital; 10 of these patients had MRSA infection. Cost data was obtained by chart review and compiled into 3 categories: laboratory, antibiotic and per diem costs. Costs were calculated by summing direct costs attributable to laboratory tests and equipment, antibiotic use, and days of hospital stay attributable to *S. aureus* infection. Total costs in these categories were compared between MRSA and methicillin-sensitive *S. aureus* (MSSA) infections by analysis of variance (ANOVA), and the mean cost attributable to MRSA infection was significantly higher than MSSA infection (USD 7,481 vs. USD 2,377, p < 0.001). While the study was small in size, it suggested there were significant differences in the costs associated with MRSA and MSSA infections.

In 1999, Rubin et al. [13] performed one of the largest studies to date addressing the issue of higher costs associated with MRSA infection. This study utilized an administrative database to obtain cases of *S. aureus* infection, including bloodstream infections, pneumonia, endocarditis and surgical site infections. While the use of administrative data was innovative, several assumptions were made which significantly limit the results. Any missing information in the data set was artificially estimated by a 'clinical panel' of 4 infectious disease physicians. For example, the database did not specifically differentiate between MRSA and MSSA infections, so the clinical panel estimated the differences in resource use between MRSA and MSSA patients and applied that difference to the average cost of a *S. aureus* infection, which was available. 13,550 cases of *S. aureus* infection were included in the analysis. The attributable cost of a MRSA infection was estimated to be USD 2,500 more than that of MSSA (USD 34,000 vs. USD 31,500). The authors noted their cost estimate was approximate, and further study was needed.

Other MRSA cost studies have performed only crude assessments. Kim et al. [14] examined the expense of controlling MRSA in an urban university hospital. Both MRSA-infected and MRSA-colonized patients were included in the study. For MRSA-infected patients, costs attributable to MRSA infection were determined by calculating the days of hospitalization attributable to infection, using the Appropriateness Evaluation Protocol [15]. All costs for days during a MRSA hospitalization were considered attributable to MRSA. For patients who were MRSA-colonized without infection, the impact of MRSA was calculated using the cost of isolation for the total number of days spent in contact isolation. There were 20 patients with MRSA infection, and the mean attributable cost of MRSA infection for these patients was USD 14,360. Seventy-nine patients were colonized with MRSA but not infected, and the estimated mean cost of isolation was USD 1,363 per admission. The main limitations of this analysis were the small sample size and the lack of a control group for statistical comparisons.

McHugh and Riley [4] examined the cost and risk factors of MRSA bloodstream infection using a 1:2 case-control design. Hospitalized patients with MSSA bloodstream infection served as controls. Non-parametric univariate tests were used for comparisons of cost estimates. An attempt was made to control for severity of illness in the analysis by stratifying by the Case Mix Index. For patients with a Case Mix Index ≤2 (lower severity of illness), costs per patient day between MRSA and MSSA patients were not different (USD 2,715 vs. USD 2,462, respectively). However, for patients with a Case Mix Index >2, MRSA cost USD 5,302 more per patient day than controls (p < 0.001). This study had a small sample size (20 cases and 40 controls), and no other adjustment for confounders. The use of Case Mix Index as a severity of illness measure also has not been well validated.

Capitano et al. [16] also used non-parametric univariate tests to analyze cost data in an analysis of MSSA and MRSA infections in a 375-bed long-term care facility. All patients with a positive culture for *S. aureus* in combination with clinical symptoms were included in the study. Ninety patients with *S. aureus* infection were included in the analysis; 49 with MSSA and 41 with MRSA. Only resources thought to be 'infection-related' were included as costs, based on the criteria outlined by a standardized data collection tool. Cost data for a relapse within a 30-day time period of the original infection was included. The overall cost associated with a MRSA infection was 1.95 times higher than that of MSSA infection (USD 2,607 vs. USD 1,332, respectively; p < 0.001). This study was the first to provide a cost estimate of managing MRSA infection within a long-term care facility and accounted for relapse costs associated with the initial infection.

Matched case-control studies are one way to control for confounding in cost studies [17]. Abramson and Sexton [18] performed a matched case-control study of inpatients at a university medical center, comparing patients with MRSA and MSSA bloodstream infection to hospitalized controls without a bloodstream infection. Patients were matched on primary diagnosis (determined from ICD-9 codes), total number of secondary diagnoses, age, gender and area of the hospital to which they were admitted. Ten patients with MRSA and 11 patients with MSSA were successfully matched to controls; 2 patients with MRSA bloodstream infection were excluded as appropriate matches could not be found. Hospital costs were compared using univariate nonparametric analyses. Results showed the median attributable cost of MSSA bloodstream infection was USD 9,661 and MRSA bloodstream infection was USD 27,083 (p = 0.043). While matching allowed for adjustment for some confounders, the extremely small sample size was a major limitation.

Chaix et al. [19] also performed a matched study which examined the attributable cost of MRSA infection using a medical ICU population in a French university hospital. Cases had ICU-acquired MRSA infection, and controls were patients without evidence of MRSA colonization or infection. Cases and controls were matched on age, severity of illness, and the number of organ system failures when admitted to the ICU. Due to different reimbursement methods in France, estimated costs for each patient were determined based on a previously developed model [20]. Twenty-seven MRSA patients and 27 matched controls were randomly chosen for study inclusion. Cost data was analyzed using non-parametric univariate tests, and the median total cost for MRSA cases was USD 9,275 more than for control patients. Small sample size and matched design were the main limitations to this study. The estimation of costs instead of using actual costs may also be a weakness in this analysis.

One of the major limitations of matched studies is the loss of cases due to a lack of appropriate matches in the control group [17]. Kopp et al. [21] performed a study of patients with multiple types of *S. aureus* infection in which MRSA patients were matched to MSSA patients on infection site, ICU care and age. They analyzed 36 matched pairs. Eleven patients with MRSA and 12 patients with MSSA infection were excluded due to lack of appropriate matches. Hospital costs were analyzed using non-parametric univariate tests. While median costs of patients with MRSA infection (USD 16,575) were higher than those of MSSA patients (USD 12,862), this difference was not significant (p = 0.11). The small sample size and matched design are a concern, as there was no control for underlying comorbidity in the analysis. The exclusion of 23 patients with *S. aureus* infection may also have biased cost estimates by eliminating nearly a fourth of patients from the sample.

Regression modeling is one method to adjust for confounding without matching. Engemann et al. [9] used multivariate linear regression to examine the economic outcome of MRSA surgical-site infections in a large academic medical center. Case patients (n = 121) with MRSA surgical site infection were compared to two control groups: patients with MSSA surgical-site infection (n = 165) and those without surgical site infection (n = 193). Cost analysis included any re-admissions within 90 days associated with the *S. aureus* surgical site infection. Regression was used to perform cost analyses, and the mean attributable cost of methicillin resistance was USD 13,901 per *S. aureus* surgical-site infection. This was one of the first studies to address costs associated with MRSA infection in patients with surgical site infection.

Cosgrove et al. [22] also performed a prospective cohort study of patients admitted to an urban teaching hospital. The cohort included patients with *S. aureus* bloodstream infection. Patients with MRSA were compared to patients with MSSA. Severity of illness was measured by the McCabe and Jackson score as assigned by a data collector blinded to the patients' MRSA or MSSA status. Hospital charges were collected and costs were estimated using the hospital cost-to-charge ratio. Only hospital charges following the episode of bloodstream infection were used for analysis and were log-transformed to be analyzed by linear regression. Ninety-six MRSA patients and 252 MSSA patients were included in the analysis. After adjustment for confounders in the multivariate model, including underlying comorbidities, McCabe score, and surgical procedures prior to *S. aureus* bloodstream infection, the attributable cost of MRSA bloodstream infection was USD 3,836. A large sample size, clear study design and case definitions, and multivariate adjustment of confounders were the strengths of this study.

Reed et al. [23] examined *S. aureus* bloodstream infection in a cohort of hemodialysis patients admitted to a university hospital. This prospective cohort study was unique in that propensity scores were used to adjust for confounding. Cost data included costs from the index hospitalization, as well as costs from subsequent infection-related hospitalizations within 12 weeks of the initial episode, outpatient visits and physician fees. The multivariate cost analysis was restricted to patients whose total inpatient costs could be attributed to the bloodstream infection, meaning patients were excluded from analysis if their admission was for a reason other than *S. aureus* bloodstream infection. Fifty-four MRSA and 89 MSSA bloodstream infections were included in the analysis, and the attributable cost of MRSA bloodstream infection (USD 21,251) was found to be significantly higher than that of MSSA bloodstream infection (USD 13,978, p = 0.012) in this analysis. The major strength of this study was the use of propensity scores in the regression models to adjust for unmeasured confounders. The choice of hemodialysis patients as the study group limits the ability to expand the results to other populations. However, hemodialysis patients have an increased prevalence of MRSA and bloodstream infection, and there is little data on cost of bloodstream infection in these patients.

Lodise and McKinnon [24] conducted a retrospective cohort study at a teaching hospital in Detroit, again focusing on the differences in cost associated with MRSA and MSSA bloodstream infection. Data was retrospectively collected from charts, including severity of illness as measured by the APACHE II score, calculated at the time of infection. Cost data were obtained from the hospital's finance department and analyzed using analysis of covariance (ANCOVA). Only the costs of those patients who did not die due to *S. aureus* bacteremia were included in the cost analysis (n = 273), although no reason for this exclusion was provided. After adjustment for confounding, the mean cost of hospitalization for MRSA bloodstream infection patients (USD 21,577) was significantly higher than the cost of hospitalization of patients with MSSA bloodstream infection (USD 11,688, p = 0.001). The large sample size of this study is clearly a strength, but the choice of ANCOVA is unusual and not a common method used by economists to analyze cost data.

A recent retrospective cohort study of 182 patients at a tertiary care hospital examined the impact of methicillin resistance on bloodstream infection cost [25]. While patients with MRSA bloodstream infections had longer hospital and ICU length of stay, after adjustment by propensity score, no significant cost difference was seen between the 2 groups. The difference was significant when multivariable adjustment was used: compared with ICU patients with MSSA bloodstream infections, those with such infections with MRSA had a higher median total hospital cost (USD 42,137 vs. USD 113,852), higher hospital cost after infection (USD 17,603 vs. USD 51,492), and greater length of stay after infection (10.5 vs. 20.5 days).


*Vancomycin-Resistant Enterococci*


There are fewer studies in the literature examining the cost of vancomycin-resistant enterococci (VRE) infections, although many of the same methodological issues from the MRSA studies exist in VRE analyses. Estimates of the cost attributable to VRE colonization and infection are varied, ranging from USD 12,000 to USD 77,000 (table 2).

Stosor et al. [26] examined 53 patients with vancomycin-sensitive (VSE) and resistant *Enterococcus faecium* bloodstream infections in an urban teaching hospital. Thirty-two patients had VSE and 21 had VRE bloodstream infection, and the hospitalization costs of VRE patients were, on average, USD 27,000 higher than the hospitalization costs of VSE patients (p = 0.04). A major weakness of this study was the use of the Student's t test to analyze costs, which assumes normality of data. Cost data in general are not normally distributed, and no mention was made in the study whether or not the cost data were transformed to achieve a normal distribution. The t test also will not allow adjustment for confounders, and the small sample size may have affected estimates.

The study performed by Webb et al. [27] is subject to some of the same criticisms. This case-control study was performed at an urban, tertiary-care medical center and included any inpatient infected or colonized with VRE (n = 262) or VSE (n = 157) over a 2-year period. Comparisons were made between VRE and VSE patients using the Student's t test. The case mix index was used as a severity of illness measure. Among patients with a Case Mix Index >3, differences between the costs per day for VRE and VSE patients were not significant. For patients with a Case Mix Index ≤3,

**Table 2.** The economic cost associated with VRE

| Year | First author [Ref] | Population | Sample size, n | Type of infection | Cost results |
|---|---|---|---|---|---|
| 1998 | Stosor [26] | urban teaching hospital inpatients | 51 | bloodstream | mean cost of hospitalization for patients with VSE infection was significantly less than the cost for VRE infection patients (USD 56,707 vs. USD 83,897, respectively) |
| 2001 | Webb [27] | urban tertiary-care hospital inpatients | 419 | colonization and/or infection with *E. faecium* | USD 252 difference in cost per day between patients with VRE and those with VSE if Case Mix Index ≤3 |
| 2002 | Carmeli [5] | urban teaching hospital inpatients | 880 | colonization and/or infection | additional hospital cost attributable to VRE was USD 12,766 (p < 0.001) |
| 2002 | Pelz [28] | university hospital medical and surgical ICU patients | 34 | multiple | cost of VRE infection (USD 33,251) not significantly more than VSE (USD 21,914) |
| 2003 | Song [29] | urban teaching hospital inpatients | 554 | bloodstream | median hospital charge for VRE bloodstream infection patients was USD 77,558 higher than that of patients without a bloodstream infection |
| 2009 | Butler [30] | university hospital non-surgical inpatients | 21,154 | bloodstream | the attributable costs of vancomycin resistance were between USD 1,546 and USD 1,713 |

the mean cost per day difference between cases and controls was USD 252 (p < 0.05). While the large sample size was a strong point, the choice of analysis was a weakness. The authors stated that multivariate analysis had been performed, but no difference was found between cases and controls, and none of these results were published.

Carmeli et al. [5] found lower costs associated with VRE using a matched case-control study design. This retrospective study analyzed patients with a clinical culture positive for VRE (n = 233) compared to patients without a positive clinical culture for VRE (n = 647). A propensity score was calculated to adjust for unmeasured confounding, and log-transformed costs were analyzed by linear regression. The hospital cost attributable to VRE was USD 12,766 (p < 0.001). The matched design excluded 18 patients with VRE, although adequate matches were found for the rest of this large population. The use of a propensity score to adjust for confounding was a positive feature of this analysis.

Pelz et al. [28] examined attributable costs and outcomes of infections with VRE in medical and surgical ICU patients during a 3 month period. Of 117 patients admitted, 34 developed infection with either VSE or VRE. Six patients had VRE, 16 had VSE, and an additional 6 patients had an infection with both organisms. Charge data from patients was converted to cost by the hospital's cost/charge ratio and were log-transformed to achieve a normal distribution. Cost data were analyzed by multivariate linear regression and median regression, and VRE and VSE infection were found to be significant predictors of cost in this population. However, the cost of VRE infection (USD 33,251) and VSE infection (USD 21,914) were not significantly different from one another. A small sample size was the main limitation of this study and may have prevented finding a significant difference in cost between VRE and VSE infections.

A larger study examined patients with VRE bloodstream infections compared to matched controls without bloodstream infection [29]. Controls were matched to cases on age, year of admission, days of hospitalization prior to the diagnosis of bloodstream infection, principal diagnosis and primary procedure (by ICD-9 codes), and APR-DRG (All Patient Refined Diagnosis Related Groups codes). Hospital charges were used in the cost analysis, and costs attributable to VRE bloodstream infection were determined by calculating the difference between median costs of case and control patients. From 1993 through 2000, 316 patients developed VRE bloodstream infection, and 277 were matched on at least 4 or more of the previous criteria. In this matched group, the difference in cost between cases and controls was USD 77,558, considered the attributable cost of VRE bloodstream infection. However, a significant limitation of this analysis is the lack of further adjustment for additional comorbid conditions and procedures beyond the ICD-9 code matching. The use of APR-DRG was useful as a severity of illness adjustment in this administrative database, but as the authors noted, it has generally not been well validated as a severity of illness measure.

A recent retrospective cohort examined the attributable cost of enterococcal bloodstream infections in 21,154 non-surgical patients admitted to an academic medical center between 2002 and 2003 [30]. Using administrative data, attributable hospital costs and length of stay were estimated using 2 statistical methods: multivariate generalized least squares (GLS) models and propensity score matched-pairs. The attributable costs of vancomycin-resistance were USD 1,713 in the GLS model and USD 1,546 using a propensity-score weighted GLS model. Attributable length of stay ranged from 2.2 to 3.5 days for VRE bloodstream infection cases. The use of readily available administrative data and validated coding methods are strengths to this analysis, in addition to the large sample size and inclusion of non-ICU patients. In addition, results were consistent using 2 analysis techniques, adding strength to their findings.

Few studies have examined the economic impact of resistant Gram-negative colonization or infection (table 3). Cosgrove et al. [8] studied the health and economic impact of the emergence of resistant *Enterobacter* species. In this study, all 477 enrolled patients had baseline infection with third generation cephalosporin-susceptible *Enterobacter* species. Forty-nine cases had a subsequent infection with resistant *Enterobacter*, and were matched to controls with susceptible infection based on site of infection and pre-infection length of stay. Median hospital charges were USD 40,406 for controls and USD 79,323 for cases. After adjusting for comorbidities, severity of illness and other important factors, emergence of resistance accounted for USD 29,379 in hospital charges and 9 excess days of hospitalization compared to controls. The relatively small number of cases is a limitation in this study.

Carmeli et al. [6] also examined the health and economic outcomes of antimicrobial resistance in *Pseudomonas aeruginosa*. Cases with *Pseudomonas* resistant to any of 4 study drugs (n = 144) were compared to 345 controls with susceptible *Pseudomonas*. They found no difference in hospital length of stay, mortality or costs. Using log transformed costs, the mean daily hospital charge was USD 2,059. Additional analyses were conducted to assess the impact of emerging resistance compared to baseline resistance, but emerging resistance was not associated with increased cost either.

Wilson et al. [31] looked at the direct costs attributable to multi-drug resistant *Acinetobacter baumannii* on an adult burn unit. This case-control study compared 34 patients with *A. baumannii* infection to 34 controls with similar severity of illness but susceptible *A. baumannii* infection, all hospitalized on the burn unit. Case patients had a longer length of stay, and the mean total hospital costs were USD 98,575 greater for the case patients. The mean cost per hospital day was USD 5,607 for cases and USD 4,017 for controls (p < 0.01). While this study is important because it is the first to examine the cost of *A. baumannii*, it has several limitations. The authors only examine total hospital costs, and were unable to look at the breakdown of these expenses and the drivers of increased cost in the case patients. While both case and control patients had burns over >20% of their body surface area, control patients were selected from the calendar year prior to the case patients. This difference could bias the study, since differences in practice, staffing and procedures could influence results. In addition, this method may not sufficiently control for severity of illness and comorbidities.

## Methodological Issues

Much debate exists regarding suitable study design and control selection to appropriately assess the attributable cost of antibiotic-resistant infections. Previous studies have utilized patients with antibiotic-resistant infection as cases and those with antibiotic-susceptible infections with the same organism as controls [4, 6, 8, 28, 32, 33].

**Table 3.** The economic cost associated with multidrug-resistant Gram-negative organisms

| Year | First author [Ref] | Population | Sample size, n | Type of infection | Cost results |
|---|---|---|---|---|---|
| 1999 | Carmeli [6] | inpatient with clinical culture popsitive for *P. aeruginosa* | 489 | colonization and/or infection with *P. aeruginosa* | while associated with longer length of stay, neither baseline nor emergence of resistance was associated with increased hospital charges |
| 2002 | Cosgrove [8] | inpatients with clinical culture positive for *Enterobacter* species plus antibiotics during hospitalization | 477 | colonization and/or infection with *Enterobacter* species | median hospital charges for patients with resistant *Enterobacter* species was significantly higher than those with susceptible *Enterobacter* (USD 79, 323 vs. USD 40,406); mean attributable hospital charge for emergence of resistance was USD 29,379 |
| 2003 | Stone [46] | infant inpatients in a level III–IV NICU | 562 | ESBL-producing *K. pneumoniae* | the cost of the outbreak was USD 341,751, including health-care worker time and longer length of stay for those infected |
| 2004 | Wilson [31] | inpatients in adult burn unit of academic public teaching hospital | 68 | multidrug-resistant *A. baumannii* | mean total hospital costs were USD 98,575 greater for cases with multidrug-resistant *A. baumannii* |

This method provides answers about risk factors and outcomes for the emergence of antibiotic resistance among patients previously infected with a susceptible organism, but it does not address the attributable cost of antibiotic resistance among hospitalized patients. In addition, many studies only examine the cost of resistance in ICU patients. While this information is useful, there is a need to estimate the costs of antibiotic resistance in other settings, including the community, long-term care facilities, non-ICU patients, hospital-wide and on a patient and society level. Most prior work has measured cost only from the perspective of the health-care system, using administrative records as these data are readily available. While the use of hospital administrative data is helpful, it does not capture the full cost of resistance. Outpatient and long-term costs are not captured in these estimates.

Many prior studies of the costs of antibiotic resistance have had very small sample sizes, limiting the power of these studies. Having larger sample sizes to thoroughly examine the research question of interest, increase the power of the study and decrease the standard error of the cost estimates is important. The use of retrospective cost and patient data can also be a limitation. Results can also be biased by missing or incomplete data collection. Using prospectively collected data when feasible to minimize these biases and limitations would be the optimal method. However, prospective studies can be difficult and expensive to conduct.

The cost of antibiotic resistance can be examined using several study designs. Case control and cohort studies are both options; each study design has strengths and limitations for analyzing the financial impact of antibiotic resistance. The majority of previous studies in this area have utilized a matched case-control design. This method has limitations: it requires a larger sample of controls to find adequate matches for cases, and unmatched cases must be discarded, which limits the sample size and overall power of the study. In addition, bias can be introduced if controlling for confounders is inadequate.

Use of cohort methodology can enhance the power, generalizability and application of the results. Those with resistant infections can be compared to both patients with no infection and those with infection attributable to sensitive organisms. However, if there is a low prevalence of the organism of interest, the large sample size required to capture adequate numbers of infected patients could be prohibitive. In addition, there are selection issues associated with cohort studies. Patients with infections may be systematically different than those without, and this difference must be dealt with methodologically.

Adjusting for underlying severity of illness is also important when assessing the cost of antibiotic resistance. Risk factors for acquiring a resistant infection include long ICU length of stay and prior treatment with antibiotics, which are both markers for increased severity of illness. This implies that patients with resistant infections are sicker to begin with, making separating the costs associated with resistance from those associated with underlying severity of illness important. This can be accomplished by matching patients based on severity of illness indicators including comorbidities and length of stay, or by calculating a severity of illness score for all patients, such as the Acute Physiology and Chronic Health Evaluations (APACHE II). Of note, most severity of illness indicators and chronic disease scores were not developed for risk adjustment in analysis of antibiotic-resistant infections. Different measures may need to be developed for more appropriate severity of illness adjustment in these studies.

Propensity scores can also be used to control for confounding and evaluate the model used to build the score [25, 30]. Ordinary least squares regression is one possible statistical method used for calculating the cost of resistance. While this method can control for potential confounders, it has several limitations, including the potential misspecification of the model and potential bias due to variables being omitted from the regression model. Additionally, costs must be log transformed and



Merz · Guth · Fraser

heteroskedasticity, or differing variance, must be addressed. Additional methods for analyzing cost data include 2-stage models, the use of the General Linear Model, and survival analysis.

## Cost of Prevention

Preventing transmission of antibiotic-resistant organisms comes at a price. The CDC currently recommends private patient rooms, contact precautions with gown and glove use, and appropriate hand hygiene for the care of all patients colonized or infected with antibiotic-resistant organisms [34]. Systematic screening of hospitalized patients for colonization with certain antibiotic-resistant organisms, referred to as active surveillance, has also be proposed in the USA and is being employed in several European countries [35]. The cost of these interventions includes time and energy required by health-care workers to implement infection prevention measures, managing isolation rooms, cohorting and availability of isolation rooms, and participation in educational interventions. Most infection prevention programs involve a combination of contact precautions for colonized or infected patients, use of decolonization therapy for patients colonized with certain organisms, active surveillance cultures, and improving hand hygiene compliance [36].

The study by Chaix et al. [19] examined the cost of MRSA screening cultures and contact isolation practices in a medical ICU. Costs of the infection-control program, which included screening at-risk patients at admission, weekly surveillance cultures, contact precaution, and hand washing, were computed by summing the cost of supplies, labor, and other operating costs. The total cost of infection-control measures per patient ranged from USD 340 to USD 1,480. Based on the current MRSA prevalence in the ICU (4%) and an estimate of the effectiveness of contact precautions (reduced MRSA transmission and infection by 15-fold), the authors concluded the MRSA screening cultures and isolation practices were cost effective. In sensitivity analyses, to remain cost effective, a higher MRSA prevalence on admission would be needed (up to 14%) if the effectiveness of contact precautions were reduced and if fewer infections occurred as a result of MRSA exposure.

Another study evaluated the cost-benefit of a VRE infection-control program in an adult oncology unit [37]. The program consisted of 15 different components, including VRE surveillance cultures, contact precautions for VRE-colonized or VRE–infected patients, designated nursing staff for VRE patients, and hand hygiene observations. The 8 months before the start of the infection-control program was the comparison time period for the study. The total cost of the infection-control program for 1 year was determined to be USD 116,515. A saving of USD 123,081 was estimated for a reduction in VRE bloodstream infections, USD 2,755 for fewer VRE-colonized patients, and USD 179,997 for decreased use of antibiotics. This yielded a yearly cost savings of more than USD 189,000.

Puzniak et al. [38] performed a cost-benefit analysis to investigate the cost of gown use to control VRE in a medical intensive care unit population. The study was performed during a period of active surveillance for VRE. Costs of gowns and staff time to comply with gown use were estimated for an 18-month period and were compared to a 12-month period when only glove use was required. The annual total cost of glove use only versus the addition of gowns was USD 105,821 and USD 179,816, respectively. They determined that 58 cases of VRE-colonization and 6 cases of VRE-bacteremia were prevented by the use of gowns during the study period. After accounting for the cost of gowns compared to the cost of averted VRE, the yearly net benefit of gown use was USD 419,346.

Perhaps one of the most strict prevention programs has been instituted in the Netherlands, where all patients are initially suspected to be MRSA colonized and are isolated until proven otherwise. All MRSA-positive patients and healthcare workers are given a 6-month decolonization therapy regimen, and patient wards are closed until all patients and healthcare workers are proven to be MRSA-negative. The prevalence of MRSA in the Netherlands has remained at less than 1% [39]. Vriens et al. [40] estimated the cost of their institutional MRSA-prevention program at EUR 2,800,000 over the course of a 10-year period, or approximately USD 339,000 per year. However, without this program, the expenditure associated with using additional antibiotics to treat antibiotic-resistant infections would be nearly double that amount, potentially justifying such a strict program to prevent the spread of MRSA.

In all of these studies, the probabilities of certain events were assumed. The accuracy of the estimates of the probability of transmission and infection, effectiveness of contact precautions, and cost of infection and prevention measures will influence the conclusions of these studies. There is always a level of uncertainty with these estimates [41], therefore using sensitivity analysis to determine the effect of varying these estimates with the least amount of bias is important. For example, Jernigan et al. [42] reported a 15-fold decrease in MRSA transmission for patients on contact precautions, and this value has been used as an estimate for effectiveness of this intervention [19]. While the outcome of the Jernigan study is not in question, this study was performed during the time of an outbreak with heightened sensitivity to infection-control measures. Since that time, many antibiotic-resistant organisms have become endemic in health-care institutions, and contact precautions are utilized on a routine basis. Adherence to contact precautions is not always optimal [43], and the estimate by Jernigan et al. [42] may be an overestimate of their effectiveness in some settings. Choosing the appropriate probability of events that most closely reflects the population under study should be the goal to maximize the validity of these types of studies.

## Future Directions

There are several areas that need to be studied to further our knowledge of the cost of antimicrobial resistance. Most studies currently focus on the cost associated with MRSA. There are few studies in the literature concerning the economic impact associated with VRE, multidrug-resistant Gram-negative pathogens, or *Clostridium difficile*-associated disease. Existing evidence suggests these organisms may significantly impact morbidity and mortality and increase costs. Additional research focusing on these understudied antibiotic-resistant pathogens is warranted.

Most currently available studies of the costs of antibiotic resistance are narrow in scope because the analysis is limited to 1 type of infection with a particular antibiotic-resistant organism in a single ICU unit within 1 hospital. Results from these single-center studies are difficult to generalize to other populations. Multicenter studies are needed to produce more generalizable and reliable cost estimates [44]. In addition, a great deal of health-care is delivered outside of hospitals in rehabilitation facilities, outpatient clinics and long-term care facilities [7, 44], yet few studies focus on these settings or aspects of cost. Antibiotic resistance is a significant problem for many of these other health-care facilities and further study is needed in these areas.

As previously highlighted, many cost estimates have limited accuracy and generalizability because of the study methods used. While matched case-control studies are intended to create comparable case and control groups, they may introduce bias by limiting the number of participants in a study to those who have matches and often do not adequately control for confounding. The selection of the control group is also crucial in obtaining accurate estimates, as previously described. Cohort studies may be a more appropriate study design for cost studies, though appropriate control of confounding is necessary. The utilization of propensity scores may be one method to control for residual confounding in these types of studies. Streamlined methods which are made available to others may also aid in producing comparable estimates between studies. Additionally, the use of easily accessible and uniformly available administrative data could make reproducibility of studies possible across many settings.

Large multicenter studies are needed to examine the influence of hospital type and geographic location on cost and resistance. The use of administrative databases will allow for studies with large samples sizes, which will increase study power and allow for more complex economic and statistical analysis. Additionally, long-term studies will allow for the detection of change over time.

Economic studies often require special expertise and may require a multidisciplinary approach to achieve reliable results. Expanding the traditional research team to include health-care economists and others trained in outcomes research may be necessary to appropriately analyze and interpret economic data. Fostering communication between these groups will aid in producing accurate cost analyses which will help guide future decisions concerning the management, prevention and control of antimicrobial resistance.

## References

1 Hidron AI, Edwards JR, Patel J, et al: NHSN annual update: antimicrobial-resistant pathogens associated with healthcare-associated infections: annual summary of data reported to the National Healthcare Safety Network at the Centers for Disease Control and Prevention, 2006–2007. Infect Control Hosp Epidemiol 2008;29:996–1011.

2 National Nosocomial Infections Surveillance (NNIS) System Report, data summary from January 1992 through June 2004, issued October 2004. Am J Infect Control 2004;32:470–485.

3 Centers for Disease Control and Prevention. Campaign to prevent antimicrobial resistance in healthcare settings. 2002. http://www.cdc.gov/drug resistance/healthcare/problem.htm

4 McHugh CG, Riley LW: Risk factors and costs associated with methicillin-resistant *Staphylococcus aureus* bloodstream infections. Infect Control Hosp Epidemiol 2004;25:425–430.

5 Carmeli Y, Eliopoulos G, Mozaffari E, Samore M: Health and economic outcomes of vancomycin-resistant Enterococci. Arch Intern Med 2002;162:2223–2228.

6 Carmeli Y, Troillet N, Karchmer AW, Samore MH: Health and economic outcomes of antibiotic resistance in *Pseudomonas aeruginosa*. Arch Intern Med 1999;159:1127–1132.

7 Cosgrove SE, Carmeli Y: The impact of antimicrobial resistance on health and economic outcomes. Clin Infect Dis 2003;36:1433–1437.

8 Cosgrove SE, Kaye KS, Eliopoulous GM, Carmeli Y: Health and economic outcomes of the emergence of third-generation cephalosporin resistance in Enterobacter species. Arch Intern Med 2002;162:185–190.

9 Engemann JJ, Carmeli Y, Cosgrove SE, et al: Adverse clinical and economic outcomes attributable to methicillin resistance among patients with *Staphylococcus aureus* surgical site infection. Clin Infect Dis 2003;36:592–598.

10 Office of Technology A: Impacts of antibiotic-resistant bacteria. Washington, US Government Printing Office, 1995. Report No. OTA-H-629.

11 Howard D, Cordell R, McGowan JE Jr, Packard RM, Scott RD, Solomon SL: Measuring the economic costs of antimicrobial resistance in hospital settings: summary of the Centers for Disease Control and Prevention Emory Workshop. Clin Infect Dis 2001;33:1573–1578.

12 Wakefield DS, Helms CM, Massanari RM, Mori M, Pfaller M: Cost of nosocomial infection: relative contributions of laboratory, antibiotic, and per diem costs in serious *Staphylococcus aureus* infections. Am J Infect Control 1988;16:185–192.

13 Rubin RJ, Harrington CA, Poon A, Dietrich K, Greene JA, Moiduddin A: The economic impact of *Staphylococcus aureus* infection in New York City hospitals. Emerg Infect Dis 1999;5:9–17.

14 Kim T, Oh PI, Simor AE. The economic impact of methicillin-resistant *Staphylococcus aureus* in Canadian hospitals. Infect Control Hosp Epidemiol 2001;22:99–104.

15 Gertman PM, Restuccia JD: The appropriateness evaluation protocol: a technique for assessing unnecessary days of hospital care. Med Care 1981;19:855–871.

16 Capitano B, Leshem OA, Nightingale CH, Nicolau DP: Cost effect of managing methicillin-resistant *Staphylococcus aureus* in a long-term care facility. J Am Geriatr Soc 2003;51:10–16.

17 Hollenbeak CS, Murphy D, Dunagan WC, Fraser VJ: Nonrandom selection and the attributable cost of surgical-site infections. Infect Control Hosp Epidemiol 2002;23:177–182.

18 Abramson MA, Sexton DJ: Nosocomial methicillin-resistant and methicillin-susceptible *Staphylococcus aureus* primary bacteremia: at what costs? Infect Control Hosp Epidemiol 1999;20:408–411.

19 Chaix C, Durand-Zaleski I, Alberti C, Brun-Buisson C: Control of endemic methicillin-resistant *Staphylococcus aureus*: a cost-benefit analysis in an intensive care unit. JAMA 1999;282:1745–1751.

20 Chaix C, Durand-Zaleski I, Alberti C, Brun-Buisson C: A model to compute the medical cost of patients in intensive care. Pharmacoeconomics 1999;15:573–582.

21 Kopp BJ, Nix DE, Armstrong EP: Clinical and economic analysis of methicillin-susceptible and -resistant *Staphylococcus aureus* infections. Ann Pharmacother 2004;38:1377–1382.

22 Cosgrove SE, Qi Y, Kaye KS, Harbarth S, Karchmer AW, Carmeli Y: The impact of methicillin resistance in *Staphylococcus aureus* bacteremia on patient outcomes: mortality, length of stay, and hospital charges. Infect Control Hosp Epidemiol 2005;26:166–174.

23 Reed SD, Friedman JY, Engemann JJ, et al: Costs and outcomes among hemodialysis-dependent patients with methicillin-resistant or methicillin-susceptible *Staphylococcus aureus* bacteremia. Infect Control Hosp Epidemiol 2005;26:175–83.

24 Lodise TP, McKinnon PS: Clinical and economic impact of methicillin resistance in patients with *Staphylococcus aureus* bacteremia. Diagn Microbiol Infect Dis 2005;52:113–122.

25 Ben-David D, Novikov I, Mermel LA: Are there differences in hospital cost between patients with nosocomial methicillin-resistant *Staphylococcus aureus* bloodstream infection and those with methicillin-susceptible *S. aureus* bloodstream infection? Infect Control Hosp Epidemiol 2009;30:453–460.

26   Stosor V, Peterson LR, Postelnick M, Noskin GA: *Enterococcus faecium* bacteremia: does vancomycin resistance make a difference? Arch Intern Med 1998; 158:522–527.

27   Webb M, Riley LW, Roberts RB: Cost of hospitalization for and risk factors associated with vancomycin-resistant *Enterococcus faecium* infection and colonization. Clin Infect Dis 2001;33:445–452.

28   Pelz RK, Lipsett PA, Swoboda SM, et al: Vancomycin-sensitive and vancomycin-resistant enterococcal infections in the ICU: attributable costs and outcomes. Intensive Care Med 2002;28:692–697.

29   Song X, Srinivasan A, Plaut D, Perl TM: Effect of nosocomial vancomycin-resistant enterococcal bacteremia on mortality, length of stay, and costs. Infect Control Hosp Epidemiol 2003;24:251–256.

30   Butler AM, Olsen MA, Merz LR, et al: The attributable cost of enterococcal bloodstream infections in a non-surgical hospital cohort. Infect Control Hosp Epidemiol 2009; in Press.

31   Wilson SJ, Knipe CJ, Zieger MJ, et al: Direct costs of multidrug-resistant *Acinetobacter baumannii* in the burn unit of a public teaching hospital. Am J Infect Control 2004;32:342–344.

32   Harris AD, Samore MH, Lipsitch M, Kaye KS, Perencevich E, Carmeli Y: Control-group selection importance in studies of antimicrobial resistance: examples applied to *Pseudomonas aeruginosa*, Enterococci, and *Escherichia coli*. Clin Infect Dis 2002;34:1558–1563.

33   Engemann JJ, Carmeli Y, Cosgrove SE, et al: Adverse clinical and economic outcomes attributable to methicillin resistance among patients with *Staphylococcus aureus* surgical site infection. Clin Infect Dis 2003;36:592–598.

34   Guideline for isolation precautions in hospitals. Part II. Recommendations for isolation precautions in hospitals. Hospital Infection Control Practices Advisory Committee. Am J Infect Control 1996;24: 32–52.

35   Muto CA, Jernigan JA, Ostrowsky BE, et al: SHEA guideline for preventing nosocomial transmission of multidrug-resistant strains of *Staphylococcus aureus* and enterococcus. Infect Control Hosp Epidemiol 2003;24:362–386.

36   Rubinovitch B, Pittet D: Screening for methicillin-resistant *Staphylococcus aureus* in the endemic hospital: what have we learned? J Hosp Infect 2001;47: 9–18.

37   Montecalvo MA, Jarvis WR, Uman J, et al: Costs and savings associated with infection control measures that reduced transmission of vancomycin-resistant Enterococci in an endemic setting. Infect Control Hosp Epidemiol 2001;22:437–442.

38   Puzniak LA, Gillespie KN, Leet T, Kollef M, Mundy LM: A cost-benefit analysis of gown use in controlling vancomycin-resistant *Enterococcus* transmission: is it worth the price? Infect Control Hosp Epidemiol 2004;25:418–424.

39   Tiemersma EW, Bronzwaer SL, Lyytikainen O, et al: Methicillin-resistant *Staphylococcus aureus* in Europe, 1999–2002. Emerg Infect Dis 2004;10:1627–1634.

40   Vriens M, Blok H, Fluit A, Troelstra A, Van Der Werken C, Verhoef J: Costs associated with a strict policy to eradicate methicillin-resistant *Staphylococcus aureus* in a Dutch University Medical Center: a 10-year survey. Eur J Clin Microbiol Infect Dis 2002;21:782–786.

41   Manning WG, Fryback DG, Weinstein MC: Reflecting uncertainty in cost-effectiveness analysis; in Gold MR, Siegel JE, Russell LB, Weinstein MC (eds): Cost-Effectiveness in Health and Medicine. Oxford, Oxford University Press, 1996:247–275.

42   Jernigan JA, Titus MG, Groschel DH, Getchell-White S, Farr BM: Effectiveness of contact isolation during a hospital outbreak of methicillin-resistant *Staphylococcus aureus*. Am J Epidemiol 1996;143: 496–504.

43   Afif W, Huor P, Brassard P, Loo VG: Compliance with methicillin-resistant *Staphylococcus aureus* precautions in a teaching hospital. Am J Infect Control 2002;30:430–433.

44   McGowan JE Jr: Economic impact of antimicrobial resistance. Emerg Infect Dis 2001;7:286–292.

45   Kim T, Oh PI, Simor AE: The economic impact of methicillin-resistant *Staphylococcus aureus* in Canadian hospitals. Infect Control Hosp Epidemiol 2001;22:99–104.

46   Stone PW, Gupta A, Loughrey M, et al: Attributable costs and length of stay of an extended-spectrum beta-lactamase-producing *Klebsiella pneumoniae* outbreak in a neonatal intensive care unit. Infect Control Hosp Epidemiol 2003;24:601–606.



Liana R. Merz, PhD, MPH
BJC HealthCare
8300 Eager Road, 4th Floor, Suite No. 400-A
St. Louis, MO 63144 (USA)
Tel. +1 314 286 0371, Fax +1 314 747 3926, E-Mail lrm8993@bjc.org

Weber JT (ed): Antimicrobial Resistance – Beyond the Breakpoint.
Issues Infect Dis. Basel, Karger, 2010, vol 6, pp 120–137

# Mass Treatment of Parasitic Disease: Implications for the Development and Spread of Anthelmintic Resistance

Thomas S. Churcher[a] · Ray M. Kaplan[c] · Bernadette F. Ardelli[e] ·
Jan M. Schwenkenbecher[b] · María-Gloria Basáñez[a] ·
Patrick J. Lammie[d]

[a]Department of Infectious Disease Epidemiology, Imperial College London, and [b]Institute Biological and
Environmental Sciences, University of Aberdeen, UK; [c]Department of Infectious Diseases, College of Veterinary
Medicine, University of Georgia, Athens, Ga., and [d]Division of Parasitic Diseases, Centers for Disease Control and
Prevention, Atlanta, Ga., USA; [e]Department of Zoology, Brandon University, Brandon, Canada

**Abstract**

There has been a dramatic increase in the use of mass drug administration to reduce the morbidity
associated with helminth infections of humans, raising the likelihood that anthelmintic resistance
may become a public health concern of the future. After highlighting the scope and magnitude of
the chemotherapy-based helminth control programs presently in place, this chapter emphasizes
the mechanisms of action of the main anthelmintic drugs in use and how resistance may develop.
To date, the most established population-based mass drug administration campaigns have been
against the filarial parasites which cause human onchocerciasis and lymphatic filariasis. The molecular and parasitological evidence suggesting the presence of drug resistance in human filarial
parasites is reviewed and factors influencing the spread of drug resistant parasites are discussed,
taking examples from veterinary helminths and the use of mathematical models. In particular, the
public health impact of the development of resistance by soil-transmitted helminths, such as
hookworm, is a real concern. Implications of the development of anthelmintic resistance are discussed in relation to existing control programs, emphasizing how their monitoring and evaluation
is essential to prevent it becoming a major public health concern of the future.



Drug resistance is the bane of all chemotherapy-based control programs. Its rapid
evolution and spread can quickly render ineffective public health measures which
rely on mass drug administration (MDA), wasting valuable health resources whilst
failing to control infection and reduce the burden of disease. The dramatic and
widespread resistance to many classes of antiparasitic drug provides a warning that,

without correct management of chemotherapy-based control programs, pharmacological advances can quickly become obsolete.

Anthelmintic resistance is defined as a heritable change in a population of worms that enables them to survive drug treatments that are generally effective against the same species and stage of infection at the same dose rate [1]. In practical terms, resistance is present in a population of parasites when the efficacy of the drug falls below that which is historically expected (when all other factors are the same). Such changes occur slowly, usually over many years, and are the direct result of natural selection on parasite populations in response to drug treatments. This stands in contrast to drug tolerance, where the drug is not highly effective against a particular parasitic stage or worm species at the first exposure to the drug. Genetic data suggest that alleles of genes that confer resistance exist in worm populations prior to the introduction of the drug. The same allele that is linked to benzimidazole resistance is found in a wide variety of resistant lines, implying that resistance arose once and then spread as a neutral allele [2]. Since new mutations are not required, selection for resistance is most accurately viewed as the loss of susceptibility, rather than the gain of resistance [3].

Many parasitic nematodes have biological and genetic features that favor the development of anthelmintic resistance. Of considerable importance is the exceptionally high level of genetic diversity seen in most parasites that reproduce sexually and that parasitize mobile vertebrate hosts [4]. Short life cycles, high reproductive rates, rapid rates of nucleotide sequence evolution, and extremely large effective population sizes combine to give many parasitic worms an extremely high level of genetic diversity [2, 5]. In addition, most nematode species demonstrate a population structure consistent with high levels of gene flow, suggesting that host movement is an important determinant of nematode population genetic structure [5]. Thus, many parasitic nematodes possess both the genetic potential to respond successfully to chemical assault, and the means to assure dissemination of their resistance alleles via host movement.

At its core, anthelmintic resistance is a genetic phenomenon, but it is generally perceived as a clinical event, with resistance detected using phenotypic measures of therapeutic effectiveness such as fecal egg counts, counts of microfilariae, or in vitro sensitivity assays. However, it is important to appreciate that anthelmintic resistance is never noticed in its early stages as outright treatment failure. Survival of a low-to-moderate percent of resistant worms following anthelmintic treatment will not have any noticeable effect on the health of the host. Consequently, unless a surveillance program is in place that closely monitors the effectiveness of drug treatments over time, resistance will not be noticed clinically until levels of resistance are extremely high. This is a major problem because once resistance reaches phenotypically detectable levels, irreversible changes in the genetic structure of the worm population have already occurred, resulting in 'resistance' alleles becoming fixed in that population [3].

Laboratory-based phenotypic tests cannot detect resistance until approximately 10–25% of the worm population is resistant [6]. In helminths of farmed ruminants it is estimated that greater than 50% of the worm population must be resistant before it will be recognized clinically. It is not surprising then, that once resistance is diagnosed, 'reversion' to susceptibility is unlikely to occur. In a few instances where reversion to greater susceptibility has been demonstrated, it has proven to be short lived once the drug is reintroduced (see [7] for a review of studies investigating reversion). Consequently, to ensure the conservation of susceptibility to an anthelmintic, and thereby also ensure the long-term success of mass treatment programs, it is of great importance to develop molecular assays that can detect emergent resistance with high sensitivity in its early stages, before irreversible changes in the population structure occur and while the drugs are still highly effective.

The problems posed by anthelmintic resistance in helminth parasites of veterinary importance are not new. Resistance to thiabendazole (considered the first modern anthelmintic) was first reported in 1964 in the sheep nematode *Haemonchus contortus*, just a few years following this drug's introduction [8]. Shortly thereafter, thiabendazole resistance was reported in equine cyathostomin (small strongyle) nematodes, and then in the other major gastrointestinal trichostrongylid nematodes of sheep: *Teladorsagia (Ostertagia) circumcincta* (brown stomach worm) and *Trichostrongylus colubriformis* (black scour worm). By the mid-1970s multiple-species resistance to benzimidazole anthelmintics was common and widespread in nematode parasites of both sheep and horses throughout the world. This same pattern repeated itself in the 1970s and 1980s following the introduction of the newer imidazothiazole/tetrahydropyrimidine and avermectin/milbemycin classes of anthelmintics. By the early 1980s, reports of worms resistant to multiple drugs appeared for the first time, and presently a high prevalence of *H. contortus, T. circumcincta* and *T. colubriformis* resistant to all 3 major anthelmintic classes are documented throughout the world [9].

## Mass Treatment of Parasitic Disease

The past decade has seen a resurgence in interest in the implementation of chemotherapy-based control programs to reduce the morbidity associated with helminth infections in humans (table 1). These programs, targeting lymphatic filariasis (LF), onchocerciasis, schistosomiasis and intestinal helminthiasis, share a strategy based on MDA with relatively inexpensive drugs, but differ both in terms of their target populations and whether their ultimate objective is to control morbidity or to eliminate infection. These different goals represent distinct risks in terms of drug resistance and will be considered separately.

*Morbidity Control Programs*

Programs targeting soil transmitted helminthiasis (STH) and schistosomiasis aim to reduce morbidity by treating age or population groups that suffer the greatest disease

**Table 1.** Features of the major MDA-based helminth control programs presently in place

| Helminth infections | Major etiological agent | Organization | Main objective | Strategy | Timescale |
|---|---|---|---|---|---|
| Soil-transmitted helminths | *Ascaris lumbricoides; Trichuris trichiura; Necator americanus* | Partners for Parasite Control (www.who.int/wormcontrol) | Control of related morbidity | Regular treatment with mebendazole or albendazole 2 or 3 times a year. Integration into the countries' existing control activities. | 2001 – no date set |
| Schistosomiasis | *Schistosoma haematobium* (urinary); *Schistosoma mansoni* (hepatobiliary) | Schistosomiasis Control Initiative (www.shisto.org) and Partners for Parasite Control (www.who.int/wormcontrol) | Control of related morbidity | Treatment of >75% of school-age children and other high-risk groups annually with praziquantel. Creation of a demand for sustainable schistosomiasis control. | 2000 – no date set |
| Onchocerciasis | *Onchocerca volvulus* | African Programme for Onchocerciasis Control (www.who.int/apoc) | Elimination of morbidity (and of parasite reservoir where possible) | Annual community-directed treatment with ivermectin to all eligible populations in hyper- and mesoendemic areas for up to 25 years. *Simulium* vector control in certain foci. Includes the 'special intervention zones' of the Onchocerciasis Control Program (OCP), which finished in 2002. | 1995–2009 (APOC); 1974–2002 (OCP) |
| | | Onchocerciasis Elimination Program for the Americas (www.cartercenter.com) | Elimination of the parasite | Mass treatment with ivermectin of all the eligible population in endemic areas every 6 months. | 1992–2007 |
| Lymphatic filariasis | *Wuchereria bancrofti* | Global Programme to Eliminate Lymphatic Filariasis (www.filariasis.org) | Elimination of the parasite | >5 years of annual drug treatment to all of eligible population in endemic areas with albendazole plus either ivermectin (onchocerciasis endemic countries) or diethylcarbamazine. Aims to reduce 5-year cumulative incidence to <1 per 1,000 in children born after the start of the intervention | 1999–2020 |

burden. Community surveys demonstrate that the prevalence and intensity of infections by *Ascaris, Trichuris* and *Schistosoma* typically peak in the second decade of life. Based on these observations, a World Health Assembly resolution in 2001 called for the development of programs targeting school-aged children with treatment directed against STH and schistosomes. Operationally, most programs have focused on the treatment of school attendees. School-based drug distribution programs are relatively easy to implement and are low cost.

At the community level, parasite transmission may be reduced by school-based programs, but only to the extent that the target population is responsible for most of transmission in the community. In practice, only one fourth to one third of the total population is treated and significant reservoirs of infection persist in the community. In addition, peak hookworm prevalence and intensity are usually found in older age groups. Consequently, selective pressure for the development of drug resistance is thought to be relatively low in the context of school-based deworming programs.


*Parasite Elimination Programs*


The 2 main elimination programs, the Global Programme to Eliminate Lymphatic Filariasis (GPELF) and the Onchocerciasis Elimination Program for the Americas (OEPA) have as their ultimate goal the complete interruption of transmission. In both cases, population-wide MDA with drugs such as ivermectin that target the transmission stage of the parasite are used to decrease the availability of microfilariae to insect vectors. Although adulticidal properties against *Wuchereria bancrofti* have been attributed to both diethylcarbamazine (DEC) and albendazole, 2 of the drugs used by the GPELF, the magnitude of the adulticidal effect has not been accurately quantified, and in practice, both GPELF and OEPA aim to maintain drug pressure through MDA until adult worms die or become infertile (5 or more years for LF and 10 or more years for onchocerciasis).

The elimination strategy for GPELF is based on annual MDA with a combination of albendazole plus either DEC or ivermectin. Ivermectin is the drug of choice in sub-Saharan Africa where use of DEC is contraindicated because it may exacerbate ocular pathology in patients with onchocerciasis. The GPELF has experienced exponential program growth on the heels of a World Health Assembly resolution calling for the elimination of LF as a public health problem, the donation of albendazole and ivermectin by, respectively, GlaxoSmithKline and Merck & Co., and catalytic funding from the Bill & Melinda Gates Foundation. Programs have begun in more than 40 of the 80 countries where LF is endemic and, counting India where DEC is used (for the most part without co-administered albendazole), 600 million persons are under treatment, nearly half of the world's at-risk population [10].

OEPA's strategy is based on ivermectin treatment twice per year. Thirteen foci of infection remain, with about 500,000 persons at risk. Several foci seem to be on the

   Churcher · Kaplan · Ardelli · Schwenkenbecher · Basáñez · Lammie

verge of extinction as assessed by monitoring of infection in *Simulium* vectors and the absence of seroconversion in children [11]. At present, onchocerciasis in many parts of Africa is not considered to be an eliminable infection, as mathematical models indicate that under current treatment frequency (yearly), coverage levels and efficient vectors, it may be necessary to treat for up to 35 years to eliminate the parasite from highly endemic areas [12].

As elimination programs, both GPELF and OEPA strive to achieve high coverage (70 and 85%, respectively) of the population; consequently, therapeutic benefits are provided to a large proportion of persons. As a result, significant declines in microfilarial prevalence and intensity, as well as transmission have been observed following repeated cycles of MDA. Additional collateral public health benefits have been observed in LF programs that distributed albendazole. After 2 cycles of MDA, hookworm prevalence and intensity declined by more than 85%, smaller decreases were observed for *Ascaris* and *Trichuris* [13]. Ivermectin is also known to have effects on intestinal helminths; however, there are few published data that document the impact of the effect of ivermectin on STH when the drug is used in the programmatic context. From the biological perspective, however, the risk that non-targeted STH species will develop drug resistance is certainly greater because of their shorter generation times. The danger is that while trying to control one parasite, drug resistance may develop undetected in another species. With this in mind, the recent global effort to integrate the control of neglected tropical diseases [14] should consider integrating their drug efficacy monitoring in addition to their treatment delivery mechanisms.


## Summary of Main Mechanisms of Action in Anthelmintics

*Drugs Which Target Ligand-Gated Ion Channels*

Nicotinic acetylcholine (nAch), serotonin (5-HT$_3$, MOD-1), gamma-aminobutyric acid (GABA$_A$), glycine, histamine-gated and glutamate-gated chloride receptors (GluCl) are all ligand-gated ion channels that comprise the cys loop superfamily of receptors. These ion channels form pores in the parasite cell membrane and their receptors are often targets of anthelmintics. The anthelmintics which target nAch receptors (e.g. levamisole), cause spastic paralysis of the nematode muscle that result in parasite expulsion. Macrocyclic lactones are broad spectrum anthelmintics that include the avermectins (e.g. ivermectin) and the milbemycins (e.g. moxidectin). They are thought to target the α-type subunit of invertebrate-specific GluCls [15] resulting in hyperpolarization of the cell membrane, paralysis of pharyngeal pumping and muscle paralysis. In *Ascaris suum* and *Caenorhabditis elegans*, avermectin was able to block transmission between interneurons and excitatory motor neurons, leading to paralysis of the somatic musculature. Praziquantel targets parasite muscle and tegumental membranes of trematodes, causing an increase in Ca$^{2+}$ permeability, leading to a rapid paralytic muscle contraction. Studies have demonstrated the immune system to be an important factor in the efficacy of praziquantel [16].

*Drugs Which Target Tubulin*

Benzimidazoles (such as albendazole and mebendazole) act by binding to β-tubulin and preventing its polymerization into microtubules, thereby affecting various microtubule-based processes, including mitosis, motility and intracellular transport. Tubulins are highly conserved and the selective toxicity of benzimidazole may be due to the high affinity and irreversible binding interaction of benzimidazole with nematode tubulins [17].

*Drugs Which Target Parasite Metabolism*

It is thought that DEC interacts with the host's innate immune system, as the drug has little or no activity against parasites in vitro [18]. Several sites of action have been proposed for DEC but the main effect appears to be an antagonistic action of enzymes that metabolize arachidonic acid. Arachidonic acid is produced by membrane phospholipids as a result of phospholipase $A_2$ activity on cell membranes. Treatment of animals with DEC alters arachidonic acid metabolism in both the host and the microfilariae, causing vasoconstriction, increased adhesion of endothelial cells, and immobilization of microfilariae. This allows for cytotoxic action by host platelets and granulocytes [18].

## Summary of Main Mechanisms of Resistance

*Resistance to Drugs Which Target Ligand-Gated Ion Channels*

The majority of functional studies on resistance to anthelmintics have used *C. elegans*. Levamisole-resistant mutants of *C. elegans* have been created and used to identify the genes which contributed to resistance. Two acetylcholine receptor subtypes have been identified that are associated with body muscle contraction, and they differ in their sensitivity to levamisole [19]. Evidence indicates that changes in the number or sensitivity of these subtypes may be important in conferring resistance, and similar results have also been observed in *A. suum*.

Resistance to macrocyclic lactones is thought to be associated with changes in allele frequencies for genes encoding GluCl α-type subunits. In *Cooperia oncophora*, a comparison of the 2 subunits from ivermectin-resistant and ivermectin-susceptible worms showed several amino acid differences in the ligand binding site. The

   Churcher · Kaplan · Ardelli · Schwenkenbecher · Basáñez · Lammie

function of these GluCls was studied by expressing the subunits in *Xenopus* oocytes. A significant decrease in sensitivity to ivermectin and moxidectin was observed in the ivermectin-resistant GluC13 receptor [20]. While ivermectin and moxidectin are substrates for P-glycoprotein, transcriptional changes that may contribute to resistance have not been identified.

*Resistance to Drugs Which Target Tubulin*

The most documented mutation that confers benzimidazole resistance is the phenylalanine to tyrosine substitution at position 200 on the β-tubulin isotype 1 molecule of *H. contortus* [21]. This mutation has been found in *C. oncophora, T. circumcincta* and *W. bancrofti* [22]. However, a study in cyathostomins found that the codon 200 mutation was not strictly correlated with benzimidazole resistance [23]. A phenylalanine to tyrosine or histidine substitution at position 167 is also found in some benzimidazole-resistant nematodes [21]. Various alternative hypotheses have been put forward to explain the functional significance of the 200 and 167 mutations [21, 24], though they remain to be proven.

## Molecular and Parasitological Evidence Suggesting the Development of Resistance in Filarial Parasites

At present no unequivocal cases of drug resistance in filarial parasites have been documented, though sub-optimal therapeutic responses have been reported in a number of locations. Some evidence suggests the occurrence of differential susceptibility of *W. bancrofti* to DEC and ivermectin even prior to the commencement of MDA [25]. Cases of sub-optimal responses following several years of ivermectin treatment in *Onchocerca volvulus*-infected patients have been described in Ghana [26, 27], where some individuals experience a faster repopulation of the skin by microfilariae than expected. However, it has been argued that these faster rates of repopulation could be due to causes other than drug resistance (see responses to [27]). More advanced analytical methods are required to enable atypical parasite recrudescence to be compared to the normal (pre-MDA) drug response profile, taking into consideration the variability in accuracy of techniques used to estimate parasite intensity, its natural temporal fluctuations, and the degree of between- and within- host variability.

Detection of resistance in filarial populations is challenging because for many of these parasites there are no suitable animal models and the life cycle stages have not been adapted to in vitro culture. Even if this is achieved, drugs may act together with the host immune system, reducing the usefulness of in vitro tests. Filarial species dwell deep within host tissues or are in tissues that are inaccessible for practical experiments. Thus, the most common approach for identifying genes involved in drug resistance is to measure drug-induced selection in the parasite genome. This approach assumes that the allele(s) that confer resistance are present in the population before treatment and increased use of drugs will increase the selection pressure for resistance in worms. Changes in the frequency of an allele thought to be associated with a reduced treatment response are then correlated with the parasite population's treatment history. These studies are generally not performed on drug-resistant populations.

In 1997, the Ghana National Onchocerciasis Control Programme identified 26 men and 5 women in the Lower Black Volta and Pru River Basins with a persistent microfilaridermia despite repeated ivermectin treatments [27]. Parasite material was obtained from this study and genotyped for an ABC transporter gene, *OvABC-3*. Allele C of *OvABC-3* was in higher frequency in sub-optimal responders, however, only a small number of adult worms were available for genotyping. In other studies, a number of genes from *O. volvulus* showed a change in allele frequency after ivermectin treatment. A reduction in genetic polymorphism was shown in the genes *OvMDR-1*, *OvABC-1*, *OvABC-3*, *OvPgp* and *OvPlp* in *O. volvulus* from ivermectin treated patients [28]. In different *O. volvulus* populations, 2 partial gene fragments, *OvPgp* and β-tubulin, had alleles which significantly increased in frequency after ivermectin treatment [29]. These studies, and others by the same authors, indicate that ivermectin is exerting some selection on *O. volvulus* populations, though functional studies were not performed to confirm the biological significance of these genes.

A single nucleotide polymorphism associated with anthelmintic resistance in veterinary helminths has been detected at high frequencies in populations of *W. bancrofti* [22]. This phenylalanine to tyrosine substitution at position 200 on β-tubulin was shown to be 26% higher in microfilariae sampled from parasite populations having received a single round of albendazole + ivermectin treatment than in populations naive to chemotherapy against *W. bancrofti*. The difference in resistance allele frequency between these 2 parasite populations may have been caused by prior treatment of hosts with benzimidazole drugs for soil-transmitted helminthiases or through a combination of high parasite genetic heterogeneity between hosts and a low number of hosts being sampled [30]. The significance of the position 200 mutation in filariae also needs to be confirmed with functional studies, as the presence of this mutation is not always associated with resistance in benzimidazole resistant trichostrongyles or cyathostomes [23].


**Factors Influencing the Spread of Anthelminthic Resistance**


It is easy to understand how resistance may evolve when anthelmintics are administered frequently. But what factors influence the rate at which resistance develops? Why does resistance develop so much quicker in some parasites and in some hosts than in others? We cannot provide answers to all these questions but there is much we do know. It is generally recognized by parasitologists that the most important factor affecting the rate of selection of anthelmintic resistance is the size of the unselected proportion of the population [31]. This unselected population of worms, referred to as *refugia*, provide a pool of drug-sensitive genes, which dilute the frequency of resistant alleles and this is believed to slow the evolution of resistance significantly. In practical terms, *refugia* are comprised of all larval stages in the environment (on soil/vegetation or in intermediate host or vectors) at the time of treatment, and all worms in hosts that are left untreated with anthelmintic. Parasitologists now believe that one of the major factors leading to the rapid and widespread development of anthelmintic resistance in important nematodes of livestock is the common practice of treating all animals in the herd at one time. Subsequent to treatment the only infective stages shed into the environment for a prolonged period (until a new cycle of infection and patency occurs) are from those worms that survived treatment. If treatments are given when few infective larvae are in the environment, and all hosts are treated, then eggs/larvae/microfilariae shed by the resistant worms that survived the treatment are not greatly diluted. This gives these resistant parasites a greater chance of re-infecting their hosts.

Why resistance develops more slowly in some hosts and parasites than others is a complex question which is dependent on many factors [32]. These factors relate to the parasite biology and epidemiology, the dynamics of the host-parasite relationship, and the pharmacokinetics of the drugs. Some factors relating directly to the parasite biology include: life history (generation time, direct or indirect life cycle), fecundity of female worms, lifespan of mature worms, survival of free-living stages in the environment, level of genetic diversity, manner of inheritance of resistance traits, number of genes involved, actual dose level required to kill susceptible worms of a particular species as compared to label dose level, and worm pathogenicity (and therefore need for treatment). Host factors include: levels of innate and acquired immunity, behavioral differences affecting exposure rates and differences in anthelmintic pharmacokinetics between host species. In livestock species, anthelmintic drugs generally demonstrate highest bioavailability in cattle, and lowest bioavailability in goats. It is frequently suggested that the extremely high prevalence of anthelmintic resistance in nematodes of goats is associated with this unique pharmacokinetic profile. All of these factors combined with treatment frequency, means of drug delivery (affecting pharmacodynamics and kinetics), dose rate, drug persistence, quality of drug used (e.g. expired drug) and levels of *refugia* at time of treatment interact to influence the rate of resistance development. It is difficult to know with precision or certainty how large a role each of these different factors play in the development of resistance, and most likely they change with each host/parasite relationship. However, the fact that the important nematodes of cattle and sheep/goats are extremely closely related (both phylogenetically and biologically), but resistance is much slower to evolve in nematodes of cattle, gives strong evidence that many factors other than the genetics of the worms are involved in the dynamic process of resistance selection. These factors can be modeled to measure the relative impact each has on the evolution of resistance.

## Use of Mathematical Models

The philosophy of disease control through mass chemotherapy is – in principle – simple, but optimizing its success is rather more complex and requires a thorough understanding of the biology of the parasites in question. Helminth infections typically cause chronic infections in humans and it is the intensity of parasite infection that tend to determine the severity of morbidity. Helminth infections of humans tend to have long generation times (ranging from 1 to 10+ years) and not to multiply directly within the definitive host. Humans characteristically fail to develop full protective immunity against helminth re-infection so parasite population dynamics can be represented using simple immigration-death type models, which chart the number of worms per host.

Mathematical models can provide valuable insights into the dynamics of parasite populations. Epidemiological models have been used to investigate the transient dynamics of parasite populations undergoing chemotherapy and to help optimize treatment strategies [33, 34]. They can also be used to investigate aspects of the helminths' lifecycle which are influential over the spread of anthelmintic resistance, although the scope of their conclusions remains mainly qualitative (system behavior) rather than quantitative (accurate predictions). One of the most important models for policy makers is also one of the simplest (fig. 1). The change in frequency of an allele conferring drug resistance will most likely follow a characteristic S-shaped curve. Once the resistance allele has reached a detectable frequency, it enters a period of rapid expansion, quickly resulting in nearly complete treatment failure. Evidence indicates that resistance alleles are often recessive [21], significantly reducing the time between detection and widespread treatment failure.

The majority of the early mathematical models investigating the spread of drug resistance in helminth populations have focused on parasites of veterinary importance. Insight into the spread of drug resistance in helminths of humans can be drawn from these models, though comparisons should consider how human treatment compliance, individual host variability and parasite biology may vary from that of grazing animals. Theoretical results indicate that mixing drugs with different modes of action will be more effective at reducing the spread of anthelmintic resistance than different drug rotation schemes [35]. If the resistance allele is rare in the parasite population, treating hosts with a drug dose that does not kill heterozygote parasites, but kills homozygous susceptible worms, will reduce the time until widespread treatment failure [36]. Drugs which persist within the host and prevent the establishment of susceptible parasites have also been shown to substantially increase the spread of drug resistance [36].

     

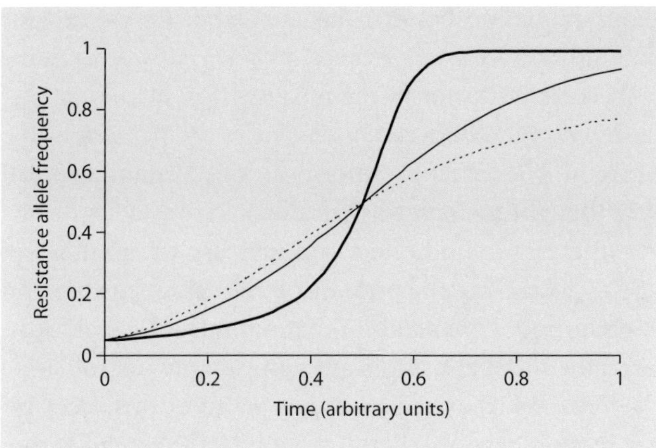


**Fig. 1.** The typical change in gene frequency of an initially rare resistance allele following selection by chemotherapy (initial allele frequency = $1 \times 10^{-2}$). The spread is governed by the equation

$$p_{t+0.025} = \frac{W_{RR}\,p_t^2 + W_{RS}\,p_t q_t}{W_{RR}\,p_t^2 + 2W\omega_{RS}\,p_t q_t + W_{SS}\,q_t^2}$$

where the gene frequency of drug-resistant and drug-susceptible alleles are $p_t$ and $q_t$ respectively, in generation $t$, with $p + q = 1$. The relative fitness of the 3 genotypes are modified to represent the relative dominance of the resistance allele, be it fully dominant (thin dotted black line; $W_{RR} = 1.0$, $W_{RS} = 1.0$ and $W_{SS} = 0.82$), semi-dominant (thin solid black line; $W_{RR} = 1.0$, $W_{RS} = 0.88$ and $W_{SS} = 0.75$), or recessive (thick solid black line; $W_{RR} = 1.0$, $W_{RS} = 0.47$ and $W_{SS} = 0.47$). Specific values are chosen so that all runs have a resistance allele frequency of 50% at time 0.5.

Mathematical models have shown how aspects of helminth biology may increase the probability that a rare, recessive resistance allele will spread successfully across the parasite population. All of the major helminth infections of humans are dioecious (have separate sexes). At low resistance allele frequencies, the transmission of resistant parasites may be impeded following chemotherapy due to single-sexed infections. Helminth parasites tend to be highly aggregated (overdispersed) within their host population, with a few hosts harboring the majority of parasites. This clumped distribution of adult parasites increases the probability that male and female resistant worms will inhabit the same host thereby increasing their probability of producing offspring.

Helminth population growth is restricted by density-dependent processes acting throughout the parasite's lifecycle. Following chemotherapy, density-dependent mechanisms constraining the transmission of resistant parasites (not regulated by the host's immune system) will be relaxed, increasing both the number of offspring produced by each resistant parasite and the spread of drug resistance [37].

Helminth parasites have a subdivided population structure as adult worms are confined to their definitive host and are only able to mate with worms co-inhabiting the same host. Parasite allele frequency can differ between hosts either due to the random nature of infection events or as a result of the metapopulation dynamics of parasite transmission. Parasite genetic differentiation between hosts has been observed for mutations associated with benzimidazole resistance present in *W. bancrofti* microfilariae taken from patients in West Africa, prior to the introduction of chemotherapy [22, 30]. Parasite genetic differentiation between hosts causes an increase in the number of homozygote offspring, a phenomenon known as the Wahlund effect. Evidence indicates that the allele thought to confer benzimidazole resistance in veterinary nematodes is recessive, so the Wahlund effect will increase the number of parasites resistant to treatment (by decreasing the proportion of resistance alleles in drug-susceptible heterozygous offspring). Non-random mating in the West African *W. bancrofti* population increased the number of resistant homozygote microfilariae by approximately 130%, which may drastically enhance the spread of this recessive resistance allele [30]. Simulation models have also highlighted how the spread of rare recessive genes is facilitated by hosts acquiring multiple infective stages simultaneously [36].

It is thought that parasite elimination (and not just the elimination of the associated morbidity) may be achievable within the GPELF and OEPA. Policymakers contemplating halting mass drug distribution should consider the possibility that anthelmintic resistance may have already developed. The presence of drug-resistant parasites will not prevent a species from being eliminated if mass chemotherapy has pushed the parasite population size beneath its breakpoint density (the mean adult worm burden below which the parasite population will tend towards local extinction due to single-sex host infections). However, the halting of control interventions before the breakpoint density is achieved will allow the surviving parasites (which may have a high resistance allele frequency) to re-infect the host population quickly. If the numbers of resistant worms manages to approach the breakpoint density before treatment is re-introduced, then chemotherapy alone will become insufficient to eliminate the parasite. Failure to eliminate the parasite on the first attempt, therefore, may render the drug ineffective for further control efforts.

Mathematical models can be utilized when designing and evaluating genetic epidemiological studies investigating anthelmintic resistance. In human onchocerciasis, it is possible to survey adult worms, microfilariae and infective larvae. However, facets of *O. volvulus*'s biology, the different life-expectancies of the parasite life-stages, and the pharmacodynamic properties of ivermectin will cause the resistance allele frequency to vary over time and across the different parasite life-stages [37]. Genetic epidemiological surveys should carefully consider which life-stage to sample, and the time points following treatment at which these samples should be taken. Sampling schemes should also reflect the parasite's aggregated distribution among the host population and account for possible variations in parasite resistance allele frequency in the hosts that are sampled. Ideally, genetically structured mathematical models should be developed and used to explore the possible spread of anthelmintic resistance for each of the different helminth infections of humans and guide the monitoring and evaluation of genetic epidemiological surveys.

**Hookworm: Does Resistance Already Exist?**

Hookworms are intestinal parasitic nematodes belonging to the group of soil-transmitted helminths. The two species infecting humans are *Necator americanus* and *Ancylostoma duodenale*. Hookworms are the second most common human helminthiasis, infecting an estimated 1.3 billion people worldwide. The significant morbidity in human populations caused by hookworm can be controlled by periodic chemotherapy using drugs. While a number of anthelmintic drugs are effective against hookworms, the most commonly used agents for treatment of hookworm disease are albendazole and mebendazole of the benzimidazole class, because they are available at low cost and easily given to people as single-dose tablets in MDA. Some MDA using benzimidazoles were aimed directly against human gut nematodes. However, the main impact on intestinal helminths appears to be due to the addition of benzimidazole to the drugs used in the GPELF [12].

Significant drug resistance has been observed in hookworm-related strongyle worms in veterinary studies, where the extensive use of benzimidazole- and avermectin-based drugs selected resistant genotypes of parasites like *H. contortus*, which threatens the small ruminant industries in many countries. Cases of reduced levels of treatment efficacy of human hookworm infection have been reported for mebendazole in Mali [38] and for pyrantel in Australia [39], although these cases fall short of conclusive evidence due to methodological weaknesses. Reduced sensitivity of hookworm has been reported in eggs recovered from children on Pemba Island (Tanzania) who have been exposed to treatment with benzimidazole over a period of 5 years [40]. However, it was not possible to conclude that a drug-resistant hookworm population had been built up because the presence of hookworm strains with different susceptibility prior to the introduction of chemotherapy could not be ruled out. Since confirmatory controlled drug efficacy experiments carried out with animals in veterinary practice cannot be performed with human subjects, reliable tests for the diagnosis of drug resistance in gut nematodes are needed. Recently, egg hatch assays have been adapted from veterinary practice and refined for the field testing of developing resistance to benzimidazole, and a larval motility assay appears to detect resistance to ivermectin [6]. To date, the only study which investigated the relationship between anthelmintic resistance in hookworms and genetic polymorphisms found no association between specific alleles and resistance [41]. However, this study focused on codon 200 of the β-tubulin gene, while mutations in codon 167 and in other positions related to benzimidazole resistance remain to be investigated in these worms. Moreover, one can assume that mutations in other β-tubulin isotypes or microtubule-associated proteins provide alternative mechanisms contributing to resistance to benzimidazole. Thus, the subject of developing resistance of hookworms to benzimidazole and other drugs remains an important part of public health surveys and a highly challenging field of research.

## Conclusions

Due to high pre-control parasite endemicity, long lifespan of reproductive adult worms, pharmacodynamic properties of anthelmintic drugs, and resilience of parasite populations to control perturbations, chemotherapy-based control programs are expected to require many years of regular treatment in order to achieve their objectives. With so many people receiving, and predicted to receive, treatment for such an extended period, the selective pressure for the development of anthelmintic resistance is immense. However, the public health significance that any anthelmintic resistance (present before the intervention, or developing after its inception) may have on the success of the control programs, is by no means predetermined. Praziquantel has been used to control schistosomiasis at the community level for a prolonged period in Egypt and yet there are no reported cases of widespread treatment failure, even in areas where individuals previously failed to respond to treatment [42].

The exclusive reliance of human helminth control programs on single drugs makes the control of these diseases highly vulnerable to anthelmintic resistance. Ivermectin is the only drug which can be feasible used for the safe mass treatment of human onchocerciasis. Schistosomiasis control is wholly dependent on the drug praziquantel, and intestinal nematode treatment is reliant on albendazole, mebendazole and, to some extent, pyrantel and levamisole. The relative importance of resistance to a particular drug class needs to be appreciated in the context of what can be expected in the future with regard to development and marketing of new anthelmintics (meaning completely new drug classes, not just new products of existing classes). Unlike most therapeutics that are developed first for humans and only then later used in animals when costs are reduced, anthelmintics are developed for the veterinary market, and then later used in humans. However, in the past 20 years, there has been limited investment in antiparasitic discovery by pharmaceutical companies, and the current trend is toward declining investment in research and development [43]. The great cost associated with the development of new drugs and the modest size of the anthelmintic market, have created an environment in which few animal health companies are committed to the discovery of new antiparasitic drugs. Thus, it is most probable that the development of resistance will continue to outpace the introduction of new anthelmintic drugs, and therefore, the management and prevention of resistance will become increasingly important.

The development of drug resistance to any parasite could derail parasite control and elimination and have negative consequences for other control programs as well as taking an effective tool out of the anti-parasite armamentarium and reducing political support for other elimination programs. Few programs are conducting surveillance to monitor therapeutic responses to MDA, nor are the relationships between coverage, systematic non-compliance and changes in parasite allele frequency of possible resistance markers being rigorously addressed. We may also need to consider alternative strategies, such as using new drug combinations or rotating drugs, in order to maintain the effectiveness of the tools we have. The risk of drug resistance hampering helminth elimination efforts may be reduced by supplementing MDA with other transmission-control measures. For example, vector control could be added to indirectly transmitted helminth control programs as the parasite nears elimination and the risk of resistant worm transmission increases.

To avoid the negative consequences of the development of drug resistance, surveillance and research are critical. In the absence of sensitive phenotypic tests to detect the emergence of anthelmintic resistance, it is of great importance to develop sensitive molecular assays which can identify drug resistance before it becomes a major public health concern. Unfortunately, the knowledge needed to develop such assays for nematode parasites of humans is woefully deficient. Research into molecular mechanisms of resistance therefore needs to be made a priority, so that the emergence of resistant genotypes can be properly monitored in areas where anthelmintic mass treatment programs are being implemented. Gene polymorphisms are not always adequate to describe or account for drug resistance as these can vary with strain genotype and drug concentration. Many pathogens utilize alternative mechanisms involving gene regulation to bypass drug effects. These mechanisms may involve over-expression of transporter(s) in response to drugs, induction of alternative pathways to circumvent drug toxicity or down-regulation of targets that enhance drug toxicity. These mechanisms have not been explored in helminths and warrant investigation. Future investigations on resistance mechanisms should avoid estimations of drug selection on a gene-by-gene basis and should shift in focus from single genes to gene networks or genomes, and from gene-structure to gene-regulation.

With this in mind, the global helminth control programs currently looking to expand the use of MDA should ensure that sufficient parasites are collected from around the world in order to provide a genetic historical (baseline) record which can be referred to in decades to come if mass chemotherapy becomes widespread. Helminth control programs should consider the possibility of anthelmintic resistance from the outset and place their monitoring and evaluation activities within the context of strong population biology and mathematical epidemiology.

## References


1 Prichard RK, Hall CA, Kelly JD, Martin IC, Donald AD: The problem of anthelmintic resistance in nematodes. Aust Vet J 1980;56:239–251.

2 Anderson TJC, Blouin MS, Beech RN: Population biology of parasitic nematodes: applications of genetic markers. Adv Parasitol 1998;41:219–283.

3 Roos MH, Kwa MSG, Grant WN: New genetic and practical implications of selection for anthelmintic resistance in parasitic nematodes. Parasitol Today 1995;11:148–150.

4 Blouin MS: Mitochondrial DNA diversity in nematodes. J Helminthol 1998;72:285–289.

5 Blouin MS, Yowell CA, Courtney CH, Dame JB: Host movement and the genetic structure of populations of parasitic nematodes. Genetics 1995;141:1007–1014.

6 Kotze AC, Coleman GT, Mai A, McCarthy JS: Field evaluation of anthelmintic drug sensitivity using in vitro egg hatch and larval motility assays with *Necator americanus* recovered from human clinical isolates. Int J Parasitol 2005;35:445–453.

7 Jackson F, Coop R: The development of anthelmintic resistance in sheep nematodes. Parasitology 2000;120:S95–S107.

8   Conway DP: Variance in effectiveness of thiabendazole against *Haemonchus contortus* in sheep. Am J Vet Res 1964;25:844–845.

9   Kaplan RM: Drug resistance in nematodes of veterinary importance: a status report. Trends Parasitol 2004;20:477–481.

10  World Health Organization: Weekly Epidemiological Review, 2 June, No. 22. Geneva, WHO, 2006, pp 221–232.

11  Gomez-Priego A, Mendoza R, de-la-Rosa JL: Prevalence of antibodies to *Onchocerca volvulus* in residents of Oaxaca, Mexico, treated for 10 years with ivermectin. Clin Diagn Lab Immun 2005;12: 40–43.

12  Winnen M, Plaisier AP, Alley ES, Nagelkerke NJ, van Oortmarssen G, Boatin BA, Habbema JD: Can ivermectin mass treatments eliminate onchocerciasis in Africa? B World Health Organ 2002;80:384–391.

13  Oqueka T, Supali T, Ismid IS, Purnomo, Ruckert P, Bradley M, Fischer P: Impact of two rounds of mass drug administration using diethylcarbamazine combined with albendazole on the prevalence of *Brugia timori* and of intestinal helminths on Alor Island, Indonesia. Filaria J 2005;4:5.

14  Hotez PJ, Molyneux DH, Fenwick A, Ottesen E, Ehrlich Sachs S, Sachs JD: Incorporating a rapid-impact package for neglected tropical diseases with programs for HIV/AIDS, tuberculosis, and malaria. PLoS Med 2006;3:e102.

15  Cully DF, Vassilatis DK, Liu KK, Paress PS, Vanderploeg LHT, Schaeffer JM, Arena JP: Cloning of an avermectin-sensitive glutamate-gated chloride channel from *Caenorhabditis elegans*. Nature 1994; 371:707–711.

16  Harnett W, Kusel JR: Increased exposure of parasite antigens at the surface of adult male *Schistosoma mansoni* exposed to praziquantel in vitro. Parasitology 1986;93:401–405.

17  Lacey E: The role of the cytoskeletal protein, tubulin, in the mode of action and mechanism of drug-resistance to benzimidazoles. Int J Parasitol 1988;18: 885–936.

18  Maizels RM, Denham DA: Diethylcarbamazine (DEC): immunopharmacological interactions of an anti-filarial drug. Parasitology 1992;105:S49–S60

19  Martin RJ, Bai GX, Clark CL, Robertson AP: Methyridine (2-[2-methoxyethyl]-pyridine) and levamisole activate different ACh receptor subtypes in nematode parasites: a new lead for levamisole-resistance. Brit J Pharmacol 2003;140:1068–1076.

20  Njue AI, Prichard RK: Genetic variability of glutamate-gated chloride channel genes in ivermectin-susceptible and -resistant strains of *Cooperia oncophora*. Parasitology 2004;129:741–751.

21  Prichard RK: Genetic variability following selection of *Haemonchus contortus* with anthelmintics. Trends Parasitol 2001;17:445–453.

22  Schwab AE, Boakye DA, Kyelem D, Prichard RK: Detection of benzimidazole resistance-associated mutations in the filarial nematode *Wuchereria bancrofti* and evidence for selection by albendazole and ivermectin combination treatment. Am J Trop Med Hyg 2005;73:234–238.

23  Drogemuller M, Failing K, Schnieder T, von Samson-Himmelstjerna G: Effect of repeated benzimidazole treatments with increasing dosages on the phenotype of resistance and the beta-tubulin codon 200 genotype distribution in a benzimidazole-resistant cyathostomin population. Vet Parasitol 2004;123:201–213.

24  Robinson MW, McFerran N, Trudgett A, Hoey L, Fairweather I: A possible model of benzimidazole binding to beta-tubulin disclosed by invoking an inter-domain movement. J Mol Graph Model 2004; 23:275–284.

25  Eberhard ML, Lammie PJ, Dickinson CM, Roberts JM: Evidence of nonsusceptibility to diethylcarbamazine in *Wuchereria bancrofti*. J Infect Dis 1991; 163:1157–1160.

26  Awadzi K, Attah SK, Addy ET, Opoku NO, Quartey BT, Lazdins-Helds JK, Ahmed K, Boatin BA, Boakye DA, Edwards G: Thirty-month follow-up of suboptimal responders to multiple treatments with ivermectin, in two onchocerciasis-endemic foci in Ghana. Ann Trop Med Parasit 2004;98:359–370.

27  Osei-Atweneboana MY, Eng JK, Boakye DA, Gyapong JO, Prichard RK: Prevalence and intensity of *Onchocerca volvulus* infection and efficacy of ivermectin in endemic communities in Ghana: a two-phase epidemiological study. Lancet. 2007;369: 2021–2029.

28  Ardelli BF, Guerriero SB, Prichard RK: Ivermectin imposes selection pressure on P-glycoprotein from *Onchocerca volvulus*: linkage disequilibrium and genotype diversity. Parasitology 2006;132:375–386.

29  Eng JKL, Prichard RK: A comparison of genetic polymorphism in populations of *Onchocerca volvulus* from untreated- and ivermectin-treated patients. Mol Biochem Parasit 2005;142:193–202.

30  Churcher TS; Schwab AE; Prichard RK; Basáñez MG: An Analysis of genetic diversity and inbreeding in *Wuchereria bancrofti*: implications for the spread and detection of drug resistance. PLoS NTD 2008;2:e211

31  Van Wyk JA: Refugia: overlooked as perhaps the most potent factor concerning the development of anthelmintic resistance. Onderstepoort J Vet Res 2001;68:55–67.


   Churcher · Kaplan · Ardelli · Schwenkenbecher · Basáñez · Lammie

32  Sangster NC, Dobson RJ: Anthelmintic resistance; in: Lee DL (ed): The Biology of Nematodes. London, Taylor & Francis, 2002, pp 531–567.

33  Subramanian S, Stolk WA, Ramaiah KD, Plaisier AP, Krishnamoorthy K, Van Oortmarssen GJ, Dominic Amalraj D, Habbema JD, Das PK: The dynamics of *Wuchereria bancrofti* infection: a model-based analysis of longitudinal data from Pondicherry, India. Parasitology 2004;128:467–482.

34  Filipe JA, Boussinesq M, Renz A, Collins RC, Vivas-Martinez S, Grillet ME, Little MP, Basáñez MG: Human infection patterns and heterogeneous exposure in river blindness. Proc Natl Acad Sci USA 2005; 102:15265–15270.

35  Barnes EH, Dobson RJ, Barger IA: Worm control and anthelmintic resistance: adventures with a model. Parasitol Today 1995;11:56–63.

36  Smith G, Grenfell BT, Isham V, Cornell S: Anthelmintic resistance revisited: under-dosing, chemoprophylactic strategies, and mating probabilities. Int J Parasitol 1999;29:77–91.

37  Churcher TS; Basáñez MG: Density dependence and the spread of anthelmintic resistance. Evolution 2008;62:528–537.

38  De Clercq D, Sacko M, Behnke J, Gilbert F, Dorny P, Vercruysse J: Failure of mebendazole in treatment of human hookworm infections in the southern region of Mali. Am J Trop Med Hyg 1997;57:25–30.

39  Reynoldson JA, Behnke JM, Pallant LJ, Macnish MG, Gilbert F, Giles S, Spargo RJ, Thompson RC: Failure of pyrantel in treatment of human hookworm infections (*Ancylostoma duodenale*) in the Kimberley region of north west Australia. Acta Trop 1997;68:301–312.

40  Albonico M, Wright V, Ramsan M, Haji HJ, Taylor M, Savioli L, Bickle Q: Development of the egg hatch assay for detection of anthelminthic resistance in human hookworms. Int J Parasitol 2005;35:803–811.

41  Albonico M, Wright V, Bickle Q: Molecular analysis of the beta-tubulin gene of human hookworms as a basis for possible benzimidazole resistance on Pemba Island. Mol Biochem Parasit 2004;134:281–284.

42  Botros S, Sayed H, Amer N, El-Ghannam M, Bennett JL, Day TA: Current status of sensitivity to praziquantel in a focus of potential drug resistance in Egypt. Int J Parasitol 2005;35:787–791.

43  Geary TG, Conder GA, Bishop B: The changing landscape of antiparasitic drug discovery for veterinary medicine. Trends Parasitol 2004;20:449–455.

Thomas S. Churcher
Department of Infectious Disease Epidemiology
Imperial College London
Norfolk Place, London W2 1PG (United Kingdom)
Tel. +44 (0) 207 5943229, Fax +44 (0) 207 740 23927, E-Mail Thomas.churcher@imperial.ac.uk

Weber JT (ed): Antimicrobial Resistance – Beyond the Breakpoint.
Issues Infect Dis. Basel, Karger, 2010, vol 6, pp 138–153

# Antifungal Drug Resistance: Clinical Importance, in vitro Detection and Implications for Prophylaxis and Treatment

Beth A. Arthington-Skaggs[a] · João Pedro Frade[b]

[a]Global AIDS Program, Maputo, Mozambique; and [b]Mycotic Diseases Branch, Division of Foodborne, Bacterial and Mycotic Diseases, Centers for Disease Control and Prevention, Atlanta, Ga., USA

## Abstract

*Candida* species and *Aspergillus* species are the primary opportunistic fungal pathogens in immunocompromised patients and are associated with high morbidity and mortality. The epidemiology of invasive fungal infections is changing, challenging the therapeutic options. To date, 4 classes of antifungal drugs have been predominantly used to treat and prevent invasive fungal disease: azoles, echinocandins, flucytosine and polyenes. Large-scale surveys of in vitro antifungal drug resistance among clinical fungal pathogens have shown that emerging resistance among naturally-susceptible species is not a widespread problem; however, ongoing surveillance to detect trends in the number of infections caused by species that are intrinsically less susceptible is warranted. Antifungal prophylaxis has been shown to be effective in reducing the incidence in certain patient groups, including hematopoietic stem cell transplant recipients. Continued efforts to define specific risk factors for invasive fungal infections, implement effective prevention strategies, develop new antifungal agents, and improve the clinical utility of in vitro antifungal susceptibility testing will better position us to reduce the clinical impact of antifungal drug resistance.

Copyright © 2010 S. Karger AG, Basel

## Invasive Fungal Infections

Over the last 2 decades invasive fungal infections, caused primarily by *Candida* and *Aspergillus* species, have emerged as an important public health problem creating major challenges for health care professionals. The rising incidence of invasive fungal infections is due in large part to the growing population of immunosuppressed patients, who are at greatest risk for infection.

*Candida* bloodstream infection (BSI) is the most common clinical presentation of invasive candidiasis. Population-based surveillance studies conducted by the Centers for Disease Control and Prevention in 2 geographic regions of the United States in

1992–1993 and in 2 different regions in 1998–2000 have helped to define the burden of *Candida* BSIs. Candidemia occurred at an incidence rate of 8–10 per 100,000 population per year, with the highest rates noted in the infant and elderly populations (75 and 26 per 100,000, respectively) [1, 2]. Surveillance currently being conducted suggests these rates are increasing [3]. Risk factors for *Candida* BSI are well known and include *Candida* colonization, prolonged hospital stay, gastrointestinal surgery, use of parenteral nutrition, antibiotics, and presence of indwelling vascular catheters on which *Candida* biofilms can readily develop [4]. Among newborns treated in neonatal intensive care units, risk factors associated with *Candida* BSI include gestational age less than 32 weeks, 5-min Apgar score less than 5, shock, disseminated intravascular coagulopathy, intralipid and parenteral nutrition, central venous catheters, H2 blockers, intubation, and length of ICU stay greater than 7 days prior to *Candida* BSI [5].

*Candida* species account for 8–10% of nosocomial BSIs, making *Candida* the fourth most common cause of health care-associated BSIs in the United States [4, 6]. The distribution of species causing candidemia is changing rapidly. Although *Candida albicans* continues to be the single most common species causing candidemia, a larger proportion of *Candida* BSI in the United States is now caused by *Candida* species other than *C. albicans* [1, 3, 7–9]. The incidence of candidemia caused by *C. albicans* reported in at least 1 study (45.6%) is lower than the incidence of candidemia caused by non-*albicans Candida* species (54.4%) [7]. According to Horn et al. [7], patients with *Candida parapsilosis* candidemia showed a lower mortality rate (23.7%) compared with patients infected with other *Candida* species. Patients with *C. krusei* candidemia demonstrated the highest crude 12-week mortality (52.9%).

With regard to pathogenic molds, invasive aspergillosis is the most common filamentous fungal infection in immunocompromised patients and is a leading cause of death among hematology patients [10]. The incidence of invasive aspergillosis varies and may be as high as 11–13% in high-risk patient populations. The overall case-fatality rate associated with invasive aspergillosis has been estimated at 58%, approaching 90% in some bone marrow transplant recipients and patients with central nervous system involvement [11]. Among allogeneic hematopoietic stem cell transplant patients, the majority of invasive aspergillosis cases occur after engraftment (i.e. >30 days after transplant), and usually in association with graft versus host disease. In contrast, autologous transplant recipients most frequently develop invasive aspergillosis during the initial period of neutropenia, before engraftment has occurred [12]. The clinical application of recombinant cytokine and colony stimulating factors with antifungal therapies has shown promise but insufficient data are available to validate this therapeutic approach. Understanding the timing of disease onset in high-risk patients and the utility of immunotherapy has important implications for devising the most effective strategies to prevent invasive aspergillosis among different groups of transplant recipients in hospital and community settings.

*Aspergillus fumigatus* is the predominant cause of invasive aspergillosis, but disease caused by *Aspergillus flavus*, *Aspergillus niger*, and *Aspergillus terreus* has been detected with increasing frequency. A recent study of invasive aspergillosis in hematopoietic stem cell transplant recipients revealed a range of *Aspergillus* species causing disease, including *A. fumigatus* (56%), *A. flavus* (18.7%), *A. terreus* (16%), *A. niger* (8%), and *A. versicolor* (1.3%) [13]. Those species causing disease in solid organ transplant recipients included *A. fumigatus* (76.4%), *A. flavus* (11.8%), and *A. terreus* (11.8%). Among the *Aspergillus* species, *A. terreus* is intrinsically resistant to amphotericin B, an antifungal drug that is often used as first line treatment for invasive aspergillosis. The newer triazole antifungal voriconazole has been shown to have activity against *A. terreus*, but is not readily available in many countries. Therefore, it is crucial to identify the infecting species of *Aspergillus* and understand its intrinsic antifungal drug susceptibility pattern.

## Antifungal Drugs in Clinical Use

The majority of clinically relevant antifungal agents used today in clinical practice can be placed into distinct classes based on their fungal target: polyenes, which target ergosterol, the principal sterol in the plasma membrane of susceptible fungal cells; azoles, which target ergosterol synthesis; echinocandins, which target β-1,3 glucan synthesis; and flucytosine, which targets DNA and protein synthesis. Each of these classes is discussed below.

*Polyenes*
The polyene class of antifungal drugs, of which amphotericin B and nystatin are the most commonly used, are natural products of *Streptomyces* species. Polyene antibiotics exert their fungicidal effect by binding to ergosterol, the principal fungal sterol, in the plasma membrane of sensitive organisms causing an impairment of barrier function and leakage of cellular constituents [14].

Resistance to polyene antifungals is rare and studies have shown amphotericin B resistance, whether primary or secondary, to almost always be associated with a decrease or complete absence of ergosterol in fungal membranes [14–17]. The incidence of primary or intrinsic resistance to amphotericin B is relatively limited but such resistance can be demonstrated by yeasts such as *Malassezia furfur, Trichosporon cutaneum, Candida lusitaniae, and C. guilliermondii*, as well as filamentous fungi such as *Aspergillus terreus, Scedosporium apiospermum,* and *Fusarium* species. Secondary, or acquired, resistance to amphotericin B during or following amphotericin B therapy appears to be uncommon as 'breakthrough' candidemias in patients treated with amphotericin B are rarely noted [18, 19]. A recent study in 4 US children's hospitals suggested that amphotericin B resistance among *C. parapsilosis* isolates causing candidemia in children may represent an emerging threat [9].

Amphotericin B resistance following previous azole antifungal treatment has been described in vitro [20, 21] and in vivo [17, 22, 23] and has important clinical implications for prophylaxis and combination therapy. The basis for antagonism is thought to be depletion of membrane ergosterol as the result of azole-induced inhibition of ergosterol biosynthesis. Resistance to amphotericin B has also been associated with *Candida* biofilm production. *C. albicans* as well as *C. parapsilosis* isolates have been shown to form prominent biofilms using in vitro [24] and in vivo model systems [25, 26]. MICs to amphotericin B and to all other antifungal agents are generally many times higher for biofilm-grown isolates relative to MICs for the same isolates grown as planktonic cells [27].

*Azoles*

The azoles are by far the largest class of antifungal agents in clinical use [28]. The antifungal action of azoles in susceptible cells is produced by inhibition of ergosterol biosynthesis. Molecular mechanisms of azole resistance can be separated into 4 general categories: reduced intracellular accumulation of azole antifungal agents due to enhanced drug efflux; alteration in the quality or quantity of the target enzyme, cytochrome P-450 lanosterol demethylase; changes in plasma membrane fluidity and asymmetry leading to reduced azole permeability; and mutation of a second ergosterol biosynthetic gene, *ERG3*, which encodes the C5–6 sterol desaturase enzyme. Azole resistance due to *ERG3* inactivation has also been shown to be associated with cross-resistance to amphotericin B. Multiple mechanisms of resistance may be active in an individual isolate at the same time, resulting in a multifactorial process.

Primary or intrinsic resistance to azole antifungals is limited to a few fungal species but is well known for *C. krusei* with intrinsic fluconazole resistance. *C. glabrata* commonly shows higher MICs to fluconazole than other *Candida* species and is currently known to rapidly acquire resistance, both in vitro and in vivo, during azole exposure [29–31]. Fluconazole demonstrates a narrow spectrum of activity against filamentous fungi while the newer azole antifungals voriconazole, posaconazole and ravuconazole have shown activity against a broader range of species, including *Aspergillus* species, the dimorphic fungi, *Penicillium marneffei*, and *Fusarium* species. Azole antifungals, with the exception of posaconazole, appear to have no meaningful activity against zygomycetes, including *Rhizopus*, *Mucor* and *Rhizomucor* species [28].

Research into the mechanisms of secondary azole resistance has focused primarily on sequentially obtained *C. albicans* isolates from AIDS patients receiving long-term fluconazole therapy for the treatment or prevention of recurrent oropharyngeal candidiasis. A study to determine the prevalence of molecular mechanisms of azole resistance in highly resistant strains of *C. albicans* demonstrated that multiple mechanisms were acting simultaneously in 75% of the isolates [32]. The most prevalent mechanism of azole resistance was over-expression of drug efflux pumps, observed in 85% of the isolates, while mutation in the *ERG11* target gene, leading to reduced binding affinity to the drug, was found in 65% of isolates [32].

Fluconazole resistance among *Candida* species bloodstream isolates, defined as an MIC ≥64 µg/ml, remains low except for *C. glabrata* (9%) and *C. krusei* (40%), with studies showing values ≤3% for all other species [4, 33]. In the setting of disseminated *Candida* infections, *C. albicans* has traditionally been the most frequent cause of disease. However, recent reports suggest a trend toward a decrease in the isolation of *C. albicans* and an increase in *C. tropicalis, C. parapsilosis,* and *C. glabrata* [3, 4]. The specific proportion of disease caused by non-*albicans Candida* species can differ by geographic location both within a given country and between countries. Furthermore, the prevalence of individual *Candida* species causing invasive disease varies between medical center and patient groups with *C. parapsilosis* more common in neonatal intensive care units, *C. krusei* and *C. tropicalis* more commonly associated with haematological malignancy, and *C. albicans* and *C. glabrata* associated with solid tumors [4, 34, 35]. Although the newer azole antifungals have shown good activity against fluconazole-resistant *Candida* isolates, the threat of possible cross-resistance cannot be ignored.

*Echinocandins*
The introduction of echinocandin antifungals in 2001 represented the arrival of the first new class of antifungal agents with a novel mode of action in nearly 4 decades [36]. The echinocandins inhibit sensitive fungi by noncompetitive inhibition of the β-1,3 glucan synthase enzyme complex and thus inhibit cell wall synthesis.

To date, proposed mechanisms of echinocandin resistance include: mutations in *FKS1* encoding the major subunit of β-1,3-D-glucan synthase [26]; over-expression of *CDR*, coding for efflux pumps [37]; over-expression of *SBE2*, encoding a Golgi protein involved in transport of cell wall components [38]; and alteration in drug influx and/or efflux mediated membrane-bound translocators [39]. Caspofungin resistance in *S. cerevisiae*, mediated by over-expression of a Golgi-resident protein Sbe2p, represents a novel mechanism of antifungal resistance never before described for fungal cells [38].

The echinocandins are fungicidal for most *Candida* species and higher MICs have been observed among *C. parapsilosis, C. krusei, C. guilliermondii,* and *C. lusitaniae* isolates compared to *C. albicans, C. tropicalis* and *C. glabrata* [40–43]. Echinocandins are fungistatic for *Aspergillus* species but exhibit no meaningful activity against zygomycetes, *Cryptococcus neoformans* or *Fusarium* species. Caspofungin acetate (Cancidas) was the first representative of this new class of antifungals to receive approval by the US Food and Drug Administration (FDA) in 2001 and is licensed for the treatment of candidemia, other forms of invasive candidiasis, esophageal candidiasis, presumed fungal infections in neutropenic patients, and invasive apergillosis in patients who are refractory to or intolerant of other therapies [44–46]. Although rare, development of secondary resistance or reduced susceptibility to caspofungin during therapy has been described for *Candida* species [47–49] and suggests the potential for therapeutic failure with drugs belonging to the echinocandins, especially following prolonged therapy.

*Flucytosine*

Flucytosine, also known as 5-fluorocytosine, is a synthetic fluorinated pyrimidine with activity against *Candida* species, *C. neoformans* and some dematiaceous fungi. The antifungal action of flucytosine is based on the disturbance of protein synthesis and/or DNA synthesis when uracil is replaced by 5-fluorouracil in the susceptible fungal cells. Flucytosine must be internalized and processed by fungal cells to exert its antifungal activity. In yeasts, acquired resistance to flucytosine results from changes in the enzyme purine-cytosine permease (required for drug uptake into the cell), changes in the enzyme cytosine deaminase (responsible for the conversion of 5-fluorocytosine to 5-fluorouracil) or changes in the enzyme uracil phosphoribosyl-transferase (responsible for the transformation of 5-fluorouracil to 5-fluorouridine monophosphate) [14]. Most filamentous fungi naturally lack the enzymes necessary to internalize and metabolize flucytosine, explaining the absence of activity against these organisms.

Despite its limited spectrum of activity, flucytosine offers the advantages of being well tolerated, available in both oral and parenteral formulations, and providing good oral absorption and tissue distribution. Unfortunately, the use of flucytosine for primary therapy is restricted by the rapid acquisition of resistance when used as monotherapy and, therefore, clinical use remains limited to adjunctive therapy and specifically in combination with amphotericin B for the treatment of cryptococcal meningitis [50].

## Microbiological Resistance versus Clinical Resistance

The term 'resistance' can often be used to describe 2 distinctly different phenomena: the relative insensitivity of a microbe to an antimicrobial drug as determined in vitro and compared with other isolates of the same species, and persistence of an infection despite adequate therapy [51]. For this discussion, microbiological resistance will refer to the former and clinical resistance will be used to describe the latter. Clinical resistance is often multifactorial with microbiological resistance being just one of several contributing factors. Other factors include impaired host immune function, insufficient access of the agent to the infected site, accelerated metabolism of the drug, presence of contaminated implanted medical devices, as well as other reasons [52]. Microbiological resistance is objectively and reproducibly measured in the laboratory independent of clinical information and patient factors [53–57].

*Detecting Microbiological Resistance in vitro*

The interest in and demand for a laboratory test that can predict the clinical efficacy of a given antifungal therapy has driven the development of standardized reference methods for antifungal susceptibility testing of fungi. The Clinical Laboratory Standards Institute (CLSI; formally the National Committee for Clinical Laboratory

Standards), published in 1997 the M27-A broth dilution method for antifungal susceptibility testing of *Candida* species and *C. neoformans*. The successive revisions of the document in 2002 and 2008 led to the most recent version, the M27-A3 [55]. In addition, CLSI has currently standardized a broth dilution method for antifungal susceptibility testing of filamentous fungi M38-A2 [54] and an agar-based disk diffusion method for antifungal susceptibility testing of *Candida* species M44-A [53].

The Antifungal Susceptibility Testing Subcommittee of the European Committee on Antimicrobial Susceptibility Testing (AFST-EUCAST) also produced standardized methodologies for in vitro antifungal susceptibility of yeasts [56] and moulds [57]. For yeasts the methodology is similar to the CLSI M27-A3 with some modifications, including a different inoculum size, use of 2% glucose supplemented medium, flat-bottomed wells and spectrophotometric readings. For conidia-forming moulds, EUCAST methodology recommends a hemocytometer chamber instead of spectrophotometer for inoculum preparation. Breakpoints for fluconazole and voriconazole against *Candida* species have also been proposed by the EUCAST-AFST [58, 59]. This method is reproducible within and between laboratories [60] and has been evaluated with the new antifungal agents voriconazole, posaconazole and caspofungin [61, 62]. Both AFST-EUCAST and CLSI have shown to be reproducible methodologies producing similar results for in vitro antifungal susceptibility. However, CLSI breakpoints should not be used to interpret EUCAST MIC data. These reference methods have improved the reliability of antifungal susceptibility testing and provided a means by which inter-laboratory MIC studies can be conducted, novel MIC test methods can be evaluated, and in vitro activity of new antifungal agents can be assessed.

A number of commercial systems for antifungal susceptibility testing of yeasts and moulds are now widely available, including the colorimetric broth dilution-based Sensititer YeastOne system (Trek Diagnostics Systems, Westlake, Ohio, USA) and the agar dilution based Etest (AB Biodisk North America, Piscataway, N.J., USA). Both have been extensively tested and agreement with the CLSI-approved reference methods for yeasts and moulds varies from acceptable to excellent depending upon the fungal species and antifungal agent tested. The Sensititer YeastOne and, more recently, the Etest systems have received FDA approval for use in clinical laboratories in the United States and their availability has led to an increase in the number of clinical and reference laboratories willing and able to perform these tests.

While tremendous progress has been made in the field of antifungal susceptibility testing over the past 10 years, there are still important limitations that must be considered when attempting to use MICs in therapeutic decision making. For amphotericin B, broth microdilution tests using RPMI 1640 medium produce very narrow ranges of MICs precluding the ability of the test to distinguish isolates with reduced susceptibility [63]. Use of an alternative test medium, such as Antibiotic Medium 3, has been shown to broaden the range of MICs and improve detection of amphoterin B-resistant isolates [64, 65]. Agar dilution, such as the Etest, has also been shown to improve the reliability of distinguishing isolates with reduced susceptibility to amphotericin B [66].

Azole antifungal susceptibility testing of *Candida* species, especially *C. albicans* and *C. tropicalis*, using broth microdilution tests can be complicated by trailing growth. This can be defined as the reduced but persistent growth at drug concentrations above the MIC value. Trailing growth is significantly more apparent after 48 h (CLSI recommended incubation time) than after 24 h of incubation and can be so great after 48 h that azole-susceptible isolates can be mistaken as resistant. Since reading after 48 h is not normally recommended by EUCAST, trailing is not observed when using this methodology [67]. Trailing growth can also be seen on agar based methods for isolates displaying the behavior in the broth microdilution method. The incidence of trailing growth observed in fluconazole broth microdilution MIC tests can range from 11 to 18% for *C. albicans* isolates to 22 to 59% for *C. tropicalis* isolates [68–70]. Two independent studies to investigate the clinical significance of trailing growth found that such isolates were susceptible to fluconazole in vivo [71, 72]. While these data suggest that trailing growth isolates, unlike resistant isolates, do not appear to be associated with treatment failure, association with recurrent infection (i.e. by persisting below detectable levels following treatment and 'seeding' the next infection) is an important area for further investigation [73]. As the clinical significance of trailing growth is further revealed, appropriate guidelines for interpretation of this phenotype can be established.

*MIC Interpretation*

Ideally, the value of an MIC should correspond to clinical success or failure of a given therapy [74]. However, this is not a straightforward process as microbial resistance is just one of a range of factors contributing to clinical failure. Therefore, in vivo correlation of in vitro MICs is not perfect and microbial resistance, defined as an elevated MIC, is intended to convey a high, but not absolute, probability of treatment failure. An editorial on antifungal susceptibility testing states that data indicate in vitro susceptibility is predictive of the response of bacterial infections with an accuracy the authors summarize as the '90–60 rule': infections due to susceptible isolates respond to therapy ~90% of the time, whereas infections due to resistant isolates respond ~60% of the time [75]. Standardized antifungal susceptibility testing for selected organism-drug combinations (mainly *Candida* species and azole antifungal agents) can provide results with similar predictive values [75].

CLSI has established interpretive MIC breakpoints for *Candida* species isolates tested against fluconazole, itraconazole, voriconazole, flucytosine, anidulafungin, caspofungin and micafungin based on clinical outcome data of human cases and animal models of infection and using the analytical model outlined by CLSI for all types of antimicrobial testing [76]. Guidelines for interpretation of MICs for other fungal-drug combinations have not been established and therefore, routine testing of these combinations is not recommended as the clinical relevance of the MIC is unknown.

Another note of caution must be made with regard to interpretation of azole antifungal MICs for isolates obtained from pediatric cases; it has been demonstrated that azole drugs in children have significantly different pharmacokinetic parameters than in adults [77–79] and none of the data used to establish fluconazole MIC breakpoints were derived from pediatric cases [74]. In the context of recurrent or persistent disease, it can be useful to assess the relative differences between in vitro susceptibility of isolates obtained from the incident and recurrent episodes to assess whether or not decreasing microbial susceptibility is contributing to clinical failure. When these isolates are tested side-by-side, differences in MICs can be meaningful even in the absence of interpretive MIC breakpoints.

## Prevention of Invasive Fungal Infections

Risks for invasive fungal infections can be understood and prevention strategies can be developed and studied most accurately only after knowing the true burden of infection, morbidity, and mortality. To date, most large-scale and ongoing surveillance for fungal infections has been limited primarily to candidemia and, to a lesser extent, aspergillosis. While there remains more to learn with regard to risk factors for invasive fungal disease, particularly with the increasing numbers of community-onset disease cases, what is clear is that most of the identified risk factors are neither easily preventable nor modifiable. The benefits of antifungal prophylaxis must be balanced against the potential selection or induction of resistance. While there are case reports of antifungal resistance in patients receiving antifungal prophylaxis, the data indicate that widespread antifungal resistance is not emerging. Instead, resistance appears to be more specifically associated with factors related to the host, such as underlying disease and severity of immunosuppression, and overall duration and cumulative dose of fluconazole received [80].

In neutropenic patients, acquired fluconazole resistance is distinctly uncommon among susceptible *Candida* species bloodstream isolates, likely because of the shorter duration of exposure and lower cumulative dose used to treat or prevent candidemia. Population-based and sentinel surveillance data have demonstrated that in vitro azole resistance, as assessed by CLSI reference antifungal susceptibility testing methods, is relatively rare among *C. albicans, C. parapsilosis* and *C. tropicalis* bloodstream isolates [1, 2, 35]. Another study assessing the impact on resistance of 12 years of fluconazole use in clinical practice found very little variation in fluconazole susceptibility among *Candida* species isolates collected between 1992 and 2002 [80]. What has emerged as a consistent trend among leukemic or bone marrow transplant recipients receiving fluconazole prophylaxis is the increased rate of colonization and infection by the less azole-susceptible non-*albicans Candida* species. A study describing the effect of fluconazole prophylaxis on *Candida* colonization and infection among 266 neutropenic cancer patients with acute leukemia or autologous bone marrow transplantation found that *Candida* colonization and invasive disease were reduced in patients randomized to the fluconazole arm compared to those receiving placebo although colonization with non-*albicans Candida* species, particularly *C. glabrata,* was greater among patients receiving fluconazole prophylaxis and one definitive invasive *C. glabrata* infection was noted in the fluconazole group [81]. Another study of 585 cancer patients receiving allogeneic blood and marrow transplantations and fluconazole prophylaxis found that more than half of the patients positive for *Candida* colonization were colonized with a non-*albicans Candida* species at some point in the study [82]. Of the 27 patients who went on to develop candidemia, 25 were infected with a non-*albicans Candida* species and the remaining 2 with fluconazole-resistant *C. albicans* [82]. Overall, however, the risk for selection of an azole-resistant strain or species appears to be low compared to the benefit of prophylaxis in these patients at highest-risk for invasive fungal infection.

Itraconazole prophylaxis displays anti-*Aspergillus* activity, a potential advantage over fluconazole prophylaxis. However, studies comparing itraconazole versus fluconazole prophylaxis in patients with acute leukemia and hematopoietic stem cell transplant patients found no protective advantage in the itraconazole group [83, 84]. Furthermore, itraconazole prophylaxis was associated with gastrointestinal side effects and detrimental changes to cyclophosphamide metabolism in patients randomized to that arm of the study [85].

The benefit of low-dose liposomal amphotericin B for antifungal prophylaxis in bone marrow transplant patients remains controversial. Research in this field, including randomized control studies, showed no protective benefit [86], while others demonstrated a protective effect associated with low-dose liposomal amphotericin B [87]. Considering the excessive costs and common side effects of prophylaxis with this agent, its use should be limited. In another study, previous exposure of cancer patients to amphotericin B was associated with an increased frequency of invasive aspergillosis caused by *A. terreus* [88]. The increased incidence of *A. terreus,* which is intrinsically resistant to amphotericin B and less susceptible to itraconazole and voriconazole, is noteworthy although *A. fumigatus* remains the most common cause of invasive aspergillosis.

The recent introduction of voriconazole prophylaxis against aspergillosis in high-risk patients has been well-received due to its protective effect, minimal toxicity, and oral administration [89]. To date, there has not been widespread emergence of voriconazole resistance among *Aspergillus* isolates. However, breakthrough zygomycosis infections during voriconazole prophylaxis in both stem cell [90–92] and lung transplant recipients [93] has been described. Because the zygomycetes are intrinsically resistant to all azole antifungals approved to treat these infections, the magnitude of this consequence of voriconazole prophylaxis requires further investigation. Posaconazole has been shown in a limited number of studies to have some activity against the zygomycetes and its role as a prophylactic agent in patients at risk for invasive aspergillosis is currently under investigation.

The role of echinocandins for prophylaxis against invasive fungal disease remains to be determined. A few reports exist suggesting that echinocandins can effectively prevent invasive aspergillosis and candidiasis without the side effects of amphotericin B [94–97]. Ifran et al. [94] described the successful use of caspofungin for prophylaxis against invasive pulmonary aspergillosis in an allogeneic stem cell transplant patient. Another report, based on data from a randomized, double-blind, multinational trial comparing caspofungin to liposomal amphotericin B as empiric therapy in neutropenic patients with persistent fever, found that caspofungin was as effective as and generally better tolerated than liposomal amphotericin B [98]. van Burik et al. [97] studied 882 adult and pediatric hematopoetic stem-cell transplant recipients and observed the overall efficacy of micafungin for the prevention of proven or probable invasive fungal infection to be superior to that of fluconazole during the neutropenic phase after transplant. Results from these studies are promising; however, at this early stage it is difficult to predict whether or not selection of resistant fungal strains and species will occur.

## References


1 Hajjeh RA, Sofair AN, Harrison LH, Lyon GM, Arthington-Skaggs BA, Mirza SA, Phelan M, Morgan J, Lee-Yang W, Ciblak MA, Benjamin LE, Sanza LT, Huie S, Yeo SF, Brandt ME, Warnock DW: Incidence of bloodstream infections due to *Candida* species and in vitro susceptibilities of isolates collected from 1998 to 2000 in a population-based active surveillance program. J Clin Microbiol 2004; 42:1519–1527.

2 Kao AS, Brandt ME, Pruitt WR, Conn LA, Perkins BA, Stephens DS, Baughman WS, Reingold AL, Rothrock GA, Pfaller MA, Pinner RW, Hajjeh RA: The epidemiology of candidemia in two United States cities: results of a population-based active surveillance. Clin Infect Dis 1999;29:1164–1170.

3 Ahlquist A, Farley MM, Harrison LH, Baughman W, Siegel B, Hollick R, Lockhart SR, Magill SS, Chiller T: Epidemiology of candidemia in metropolitan Atlanta and Baltimore City and County: preliminary results of population-based active, laboratory surveillance, 2008–2010. 49th Intersci Conf Antimicrob Agents Chemother, San Francisco, 2009; abstr. M-1241.

4 Pfaller MA, Diekema DJ: Epidemiology of invasive candidiasis: a persistent public health problem. Clin Microbiol Rev 2007;20:133–163.

5 Saiman L, Ludington E, Pfaller M, Rangel-Frausto S, Wiblin RT, Dawson J, Blumberg HM, Patterson JE, Rinaldi M, Edwards JE, Wenzel RP, Jarvis W: Risk factors for candidemia in neonatal intensive care unit patients: the National Epidemiology of Mycosis Survey study group. Pediatr Infect Dis J 2000;19:319–324.

6 Wisplinghoff H, Bischoff T, Tallent SM, Seifert H, Wenzel RP, Edmond MB: Nosocomial bloodstream infections in US hospitals: analysis of 24,179 cases from a prospective nationwide surveillance study. Clin Infect Dis 2004; 39:309–317.

7 Horn DL, Neofytos D, Anaissie EJ, Fishman JA, Steinbach WJ, Olyaei AJ, Marr KA, Pfaller MA, Chang CH, Webster KM: Epidemiology and outcomes of candidemia in 2,019 patients: data from the prospective antifungal therapy alliance registry. Clin Infect Dis 2009;48:1695–1703.

8 Nguyen MH, Peacock Jr JE, Morris AJ, Tanner DC, Nguyen ML, Snydman DR, Wagener MM, Rinaldi MG, Yu VL: The changing face of candidemia: emergence of non-*Candida albicans* species and antifungal resistance. Am J Med 1996;100:617–623.

9 Zaoutis TE, Foraker E, McGowan KL, Mortensen J, Campos J, Walsh TJ, Klein JD: Antifungal susceptibility of *Candida* spp. isolated from pediatric patients: a survey of 4 children's hospitals. Diagn Microbiol Infect Dis 2005;52:295–298.

10 Latgé JP: *Aspergillus fumigatus* and aspergillosis. Clin Microbiol Rev 1999;12:310–350.

11 Magill SS, Chiller TM, Warnock DW: Evolving strategies in the management of aspergillosis. Expert Opin Pharmacother 2008;9:193–209.

12 Richardson MD: Changing patterns and trends in systemic fungal infections. J Antimicrob Chemother 2005;56(suppl 1):i5–i11.

13 Morgan J, Wannemuehler KA, Marr KA, Hadley S, Kontoyiannis DP, Walsh TJ, Fridkin SK, Pappas PG, Warnock DW: Incidence of invasive aspergillosis following hematopoietic stem cell and solid organ transplantation: interim results of a prospective multicenter surveillance program. Med Mycol 2005; 43(suppl 1):S49–S58.

14 Vanden Bossche H, Marichal P, Odds FC: Molecular mechanisms of drug resistance in fungi. Trends Microbiol 1994;2:393–400.

15 Kelly SL, Lamb DC, Kelly DE, Manning NJ, Loeffler J, Hebart H, Schumacher U, Einsele H: Resistance to fluconazole and cross-resistance to amphotericin B in *Candida albicans* from AIDS patients caused by defective sterol delta5,6-desaturation. FEBS Lett 1997;400:80–82.

16 Kelly SL, Lamb DC, Taylor M, Corran AJ, Baldwin BC, Powderly WG: Resistance to amphotericin B associated with defective sterol delta 8→7 isomerase in a *Cryptococcus neoformans* strain from an AIDS patient. FEMS Microbiol Lett 1994;122:39–42.

17 Nolte FS, ParkinsonT, Falconer DJ, Dix S, Williams J, Gilmore C, Geller R, Wingard JR: Isolation and characterization of fluconazole- and amphotericin B-resistant *Candida albicans* from blood of two patients with leukemia. Antimicrob Agents Chemother 1997;41:196–199.

18 Hoban DJ, Zhanel GG, Karlowsky JA: In vitro susceptibilities of *Candida* and *Cryptococcus neoformans* isolates from blood cultures of neutropenic patients. Antimicrob Agents Chemother 1999;43: 1463–1464.

19 Pfaller MA, Rhine-Chalberg J, Barry AL, Rex JH: Strain variation and antifungal susceptibility among bloodstream isolates of *Candida* species from 21 different medical institutions. Clin Infect Dis 1995; 21:1507–1509.

20 Johnson EM, Oakley KL, Radford SA, Moore CB, Warn P, Warnock DW, Denning DW: Lack of correlation of in vitro amphotericin B susceptibility testing with outcome in a murine model of *Aspergillus* infection. J Antimicrob Chemother 2000;45: 85–93.

21 Martin E, Maier F, Bhakdi S: Antagonistic effects of fluconazole and 5-fluorocytosine on candidacidal action of amphotericin B in human serum. Antimicrob Agents Chemother 1994;38:1331–1338.

22 Polak A, Scholer HJ, Wall M: Combination therapy of experimental candidiasis, cryptococcosis and aspergillosis in mice. Chemotherapy 1982;28:461–479.

23 Schaffner A, Bohler A: Amphotericin B refractory aspergillosis after itraconazole: evidence for significant antagonism. Mycoses 1993;36:421–424.

24 Kojic EM, Darouiche RO: Comparison of adherence of *Candida albicans* and *Candida parapsilosis* to silicone catheters in vitro and in vivo. Clin Microbiol Infect 2003;9:684–690.

25 Andes D, Nett J, Oschel P, Albrecht R, Marchillo K, Pitula A: Development and characterization of an in vivo central venous catheter *Candida albicans* biofilm model. Infect Immun 2004;72:6023–6031.

26 Kurtz MB, Abruzzo G, Flattery A, Bartizal K, Marrinan JA, Li W, Milligan J, Nollstadt K, Douglas CM: Characterization of echinocandin-resistant mutants of *Candida albicans*: genetic, biochemical, and virulence studies. Infect Immun 1996;64:3244–3251.

27 Mukherjee PK, Chandra J: *Candida* biofilm resistance. Drug Resist Updat 2004;7:301–309.

28 Sheehan DJ, Hitchcock CA, Sibley CM: Current and emerging azole antifungal agents. Clin Microbiol Rev 1999;12:40–79.

29 Bennett, JE, Izumikawa K, Marr KA: Mechanism of increased fluconazole resistance in *Candida glabrata* during prophylaxis. Antimicrob Agents Chemother 2004;48:1773–1777.

30 Hitchcock CA, Pye GW, Troke PF, Johnson EM, Warnock DW: Fluconazole resistance in *Candida glabrata*. Antimicrob Agents Chemother 1993;37: 1962–1965.

31 Warnock DW, Burke J, Cope NJ, Johnson EM, von Fraunhofer NA, Williams EW: Fluconazole resistance in *Candida glabrata*. Lancet 1988;2:1310.

32 Perea S, Lopez-Ribot JL, Kirkpatrick WR, McAtee RK, Santillan RA, Martinez M, Calabrese D, Sanglard D, Patterson TF: Prevalence of molecular mechanisms of resistance to azole antifungal agents in *Candida albicans* strains displaying high-level fluconazole resistance isolated from human immunodeficiency virus-infected patients. Antimicrob Agents Chemother 2001;45:2676–2684.

33 Diekema DJ, Messer SA, Brueggemann AB, Coffman SL, Doern GV, Herwaldt LA, Pfaller MA: Epidemiology of candidemia: 3-year results from the emerging infections and the epidemiology of Iowa organisms study. J Clin Microbiol 2002;40:1298–1302.

34 Meunier F, Aoun M, Bitar N: Candidemia in immunocompromised patients. Clin Infect Dis 1992; 14(suppl 1):S120–S125.

35  Pfaller MA, Diekema DJ, Jones RN, Messer SA, Hollis RJ: Trends in antifungal susceptibility of *Candida* spp. isolated from pediatric and adult patients with bloodstream infections: SENTRY Antimicrobial Surveillance Program, 1997 to 2000. J Clin Microbiol 2002;40:852–856.

36  Denning DW: Echinocandin antifungal drugs. Lancet 2003;362:1142–1151.

37  Schuetzer-Muehlbauer M, Willinger B, Krapf G, Enzinger S, Presterl E, Kuchler K: The *Candida albicans* Cdr2p ATP-binding cassette (ABC) transporter confers resistance to caspofungin. Mol Microbiol 2003;48:225–235.

38  Osherov N, May GS, Albert ND, Kontoyiannis DP: Overexpression of Sbe2p, a Golgi protein, results in resistance to caspofungin in *Saccharomyces cerevisiae*. Antimicrob Agents Chemother 2002;46:2462–2469.

39  Paderu P, Park S, Perlin DS: Caspofungin uptake is mediated by a high-affinity transporter in *Candida albicans*. Antimicrob Agents Chemother 2004;48:3845–3849.

40  Bartizal K, Gill CJ, Abruzzo GK, Flattery AM, Kong L, Scott PM, Smith JG, Leighton CE, Bouffard A, Dropinski JF, Balkovec J: In vitro preclinical evaluation studies with the echinocandin antifungal MK-0991 (L-743,872). Antimicrob Agents Chemother 1997;41:2326–2332.

41  Douglas, CM: Fungal beta(1,3)-D-glucan synthesis. Med Mycol 2001;39(suppl 1):55–66.

42  Marco F, Pfaller MA, Messer SA, Jones RN: Activity of MK-0991 (L-743,872), a new echinocandin, compared with those of LY303366 and four other antifungal agents tested against blood stream isolates of *Candida* spp. Diagn Microbiol Infect Dis 1998;32:33–37.

43  Vazquez JA, Lynch M, Boikov D, Sobel JD: In vitro activity of a new pneumocandin antifungal, L-743,872, against azole-susceptible and -resistant *Candida* species. Antimicrob Agents Chemother 1997;41:1612–1614.

44  Arathoon EG, Gotuzzo E, Noriega LM, Berman RS, DiNubile MJ, Sable CA: Randomized, double-blind, multicenter study of caspofungin versus amphotericin B for treatment of oropharyngeal and esophageal candidiases. Antimicrob Agents Chemother 2002;46:451–457.

45  Kartsonis NA, Nielsen J, Douglas CM: Caspofungin: the first in a new class of antifungal agents. Drug Resist Updat 2003;6:197–218.

46  Maertens J, Raad I, Sable CA, Ngai A, Berman R, Patterson TF, Denning D, Walsh T: Multicenter, noncomparative study to evaluate safety and efficacy of caspofungin in adults with invasive aspergillosis refractory or intolerant to amphotericin B, amphotericin B lipid formulations, or azoles. 40th Intersci Conf Antimicrob Agents Chemother, Toronto, 2000; abstr. 1103.

47  Hernandez S, López-Ribot JL, Najvar LK, McCarthy DI, Bocanegra R, Graybill JR: Caspofungin resistance in *Candida albicans*: correlating clinical outcome with laboratory susceptibility testing of three isogenic isolates serially obtained from a patient with progressive *Candida* esophagitis. Antimicrob Agents Chemother 2004;48:1382–1383.

48  Miller CD, Lomaestro BW, Park S, Perlin DS: Progressive esophagitis caused by *Candida albicans* with reduced susceptibility to caspofungin. Pharmacotherapy 2006;26:877–880.

49  Thompson GR 3rd, Wiederhold NP, Vallor AC, Villareal NC, Lewis JS 2nd, Patterson TF: Development of caspofungin resistance following prolonged therapy for invasive candidiasis secondary to *Candida glabrata* infection. Antimicrob Agents Chemother 2008;52:3783–3785.

50  Saag, MS, Graybill RJ, Larsen RA, Pappas PG, Perfect JR, Powderly WG, Sobel JD, Dismukes WE: Practice guidelines for the management of cryptococcal disease. Clin Infect Dis 2000;30:710–718.

51  Loeffler J, Stevens DA: Antifungal drug resistance. Clin Infect Dis 2003;36:S31–S41.

52  Rex JH, Pfaller MA, Galgiani JN, Bartlett MS, Espinel-Ingroff A, Ghannoum MA, Lancaster M, Odds FC, Rinaldi MG, Walsh TJ, Barry AL: Development of interpretive breakpoints for antifungal susceptibility testing: conceptual framework and analysis of in vitro-in vivo correlation data for fluconazole, itraconazole, and candida infections. Subcommittee on Antifungal Susceptibility Testing of the National Committee for Clinical Laboratory Standards. Clin Infect Dis 1997;24:235–247.

53  Clinical and Laboratory Standards Institute: Method for antifungal disk diffusion susceptibility testing of yeasts: CLSI document M44-A. 2004.

54  Clinical and Laboratory Standards Institute: Reference method for broth dilution antifungal susceptibility testing of filamentous fungi: CLSI document M38-A2. 2008.

55  Clinical and Laboratory Standards Institute: Reference method for broth dilution antifungal susceptibility testing of yeast: CLSI document M27-A3. 2008.

56  Subcommittee on Antifungal Susceptibility Testing (AFST) of the ESCMID European Committee for Antimicrobial Susceptibility Testing (EUCAST). EUCAST definitive document E.Def 7.1: method for the determination of broth dilution MICs of antifungal agents for fermentative yeasts. Clin Microbiol Infect 2008;14:398–405.

57  Subcommittee on Antifungal Susceptibility Testing (AFST) of the ESCMID European Committee for Antimicrobial Susceptibility Testing (EUCAST): EUCAST definitive document E.Def 9.1: method for the determination of broth dilution minimum inhibitory concentrations of antifungal agents for conidia forming moulds. 2008.

58  Subcommittee on Antifungal Susceptibility Testing (AFST) of the ESCMID European Committee for Antimicrobial Susceptibility Testing (EUCAST): EUCAST technical note on fluconazole. Clin Microbiol Infect 2008;14:193–195.

59  Subcommittee on Antifungal Susceptibility Testing (AFST) of the ESCMID European Committee for Antimicrobial Susceptibility Testing (EUCAST): EUCAST technical note on voriconazole. Clin Microbiol Infect 2008;14:985–987.

60  Cuenca-Estrella M, Moore CB, Barchiesi F, Bille J, Chryssanthou E, Denning DW, Donnelly JP, Dromer F, Dupont B, Rex JH, Richardson MD, Sancak B, Verweij PE, Rodríguez-Tudela JL; AFST Subcommittee of the European Committee on Antimicrobial Susceptibility Testing: Multicenter evaluation of the reproducibility of the proposed antifungal susceptibility testing method for fermentative yeasts of the Antifungal Susceptibility Testing Subcommittee of the European Committee on Antimicrobial Susceptibility Testing (AFST-EUCAST). Clin Microbiol Infect 2003;9:467–474.

61  Chryssanthou E, Cuenca-Estrella M: Comparison of the Antifungal Susceptibility Testing Subcommittee of the European Committee on Antibiotic Susceptibility Testing proposed standard and the E-test with the NCCLS broth microdilution method for voriconazole and caspofungin susceptibility testing of yeast species. J Clin Microbiol 2002;40:3841–3844.

62  Espinel-Ingroff A, Barchiesi F, Cuenca-Estrella M, Pfaller MA, Rinaldi M, Rodriguez-Tudela JL, Verweij PE: International and multicenter comparison of EUCAST and CLSI M27-A2 broth microdilution methods for testing susceptibilities of Candida spp. to fluconazole, itraconazole, posaconazole, and voriconazole. J Clin Microbiol 2005;43:3884–3889.

63  Rex JH, Pfaller MA, Rinaldi MG, Polak A, Galgiani JN: Antifungal susceptibility testing. Clin Microbiol Rev 1993;6:367–381.

64  Lozano-Chiu M, Nelson PW, Lancaster M, Pfaller MA, Rex JH: Lot-to-lot variability of antibiotic medium 3 used for testing susceptibility of Candida isolates to amphotericin B. J Clin Microbiol 1997;35:270–272.

65  Rex JH, Cooper CR Jr, Merz WG, Galgiani JN, Anaissie EJ: Detection of amphotericin B-resistant Candida isolates in a broth-based system. Antimicrob Agents Chemother 1995;39:906–909.

66  Clancy CJ, Nguyen MH: Correlation between in vitro susceptibility determined by E test and response to therapy with amphotericin B: results from a multicenter prospective study of candidemia. Antimicrob Agents Chemother 1999;43:1289–1290.

67  Coenye T, De Vos M, Vandenbosch D, Nelis H: Factors influencing the trailing endpoint observed in Candida albicans susceptibility testing using the CLSI procedure. Clin Microbiol Infect 2008;14:495–497.

68  Arthington-Skaggs BA, Lee-Yang W, Ciblak MA, Frade JP, Brandt ME, Hajjeh RA, Harrison LH, Sofair AN, Warnock DW: Comparison of visual and spectrophotometric methods of broth microdilution MIC end point determination and evaluation of a sterol quantitation method for in vitro susceptibility testing of fluconazole and itraconazole against trailing and nontrailing Candida isolates. Antimicrob Agents Chemother 2002;46:2477–2481.

69  Ostrosky-Zeichner L, Rex JH, Pappas PG, Hamill RJ, Larsen RA, Horowitz HW, Powderly WG, Hyslop N, Kauffman CA, Cleary J, Mangino JE, Lee J: Antifungal susceptibility survey of 2,000 bloodstream Candida isolates in the United States. Antimicrob Agents Chemother 2003;47:3149–3154.

70  St-Germain G: Impact of endpoint definition on the outcome of antifungal susceptibility tests with Candida species: 24- versus 48-h incubation and 50 versus 80% reduction in growth. Mycoses 2001;44:37–45.

71  Arthington-Skaggs BA, Warnock DW, Morrison CJ: Quantitation of Candida albicans ergosterol content improves the correlation between in vitro antifungal susceptibility test results and in vivo outcome after fluconazole treatment in a murine model of invasive candidiasis. Antimicrob Agents Chemother 2000;44:2081–2085.

72  Rex JH, Nelson PW, Paetznick VL, Lozano-Chiu M, Espinel-Ingroff A, Anaissie EJ: Optimizing the correlation between results of testing in vitro and therapeutic outcome in vivo for fluconazole by testing critical isolates in a murine model of invasive candidiasis. Antimicrob Agents Chemother 1998;42:129–134.

73 Smith WL, Edlind TD: Histone deacetylase inhibitors enhance *Candida albicans* sensitivity to azoles and related antifungals: correlation with reduction in *CDR* and *ERG* upregulation. Antimicrob Agents Chemother 2002;46:3532–3539.

74 Rex JH, Pfaller MA, Walsh TJ, Chaturvedi V, Espinel-Ingroff A, Ghannoum MA, Gosey LL, Odds FC, Rinaldi MG, Sheehan DJ, Warnock DW: Antifungal susceptibility testing: practical aspects and current challenges. Clin Microbiol Rev 2001;14: 643–658.

75 Rex JH, Pfaller MA: Has antifungal susceptibility testing come of age? Clin Infect Dis 2002;35:982–989.

76 Clinical and Laboratory Standards Institute: Reference method for broth dilution antifungal susceptibility testing of yeast: third informational supplement: CLSI document M27-S3. 2008.

77 Brammer KW, Coates PE: Pharmacokinetics of fluconazole in pediatric patients. Eur J Clin Microbiol Infect Dis 1994;13:325–329.

78 Saxen H, Hoppu K, Pohjavuori M: Pharmacokinetics of fluconazole in very low birth weight infants during the first two weeks of life. Clin Pharmacol Ther 1993;54:269–277.

79 Seay RE, Larson TA, Toscano JP, Bostrom BC, O'Leary MC, Uden DL: Pharmacokinetics of fluconazole in immune-compromised children with leukemia or other hematologic diseases. Pharmacotherapy 1995;15:52–58.

80 Pfaller MA, Diekema DJ: Twelve years of fluconazole in clinical practice: global trends in species distribution and fluconazole susceptibility of bloodstream isolates of *Candida*. Clin Microbiol Infect 2004;10(suppl 1):11–23.

81 Laverdiere M, Rotstein C, Bow EJ, Roberts RS, Ioannou S, Carr D, Moghaddam N: Impact of fluconazole prophylaxis on fungal colonization and infection rates in neutropenic patients. The Canadian fluconazole study. J Antimicrob Chemother 2000;46:1001–1008.

82 Marr KA, Seidel K, White TC, Bowden RA: Candidemia in allogeneic blood and marrow transplant recipients: evolution of risk factors after the adoption of prophylactic fluconazole. J Infect Dis 2000;181:309–316.

83 Marr KA, Crippa F, Leisenring W, Hoyle M, Boeckh M, Balajee SA, Nichols WG, Musher B, Corey L: Itraconazole versus fluconazole for prevention of fungal infections in patients receiving allogeneic stem cell transplants. Blood 2004;103:1527–1533.

84 Oren I, Rowe J, Sprecher H, Tamir A, Benyamini N, Akria L, Gorelik A, Dally N, Zuckerman T, Haddad N, Fineman R, Dann E: A prospective randomized trial of itraconazole vs. fluconazole for the prevention of fungal infections in patients with acute leukemia and hematopoietic stem cell transplant recipients. Bone Marrow Transplant 2006;38:127–134.

85 van Burik JA: Role of new antifungal agents in prophylaxis of mycoses in high risk patients. Curr Opin Infect Dis 2005;18:479–483.

86 Falagas, M, Vardakas K: Liposomal amphotericin B as antifungal prophylaxis in bone marrow transplant patients. Am J Hematol 2006;81:299–300.

87 Penack O, Schwartz S, Martus P, Reinwald M, Schmidt-Hieber M, Thiel E, Blau IW: Low-dose liposomal amphotericin B in the prevention of invasive fungal infections in patients with prolonged neutropenia: results from a randomized, single-center trial. Ann Oncol 2006;17:1306–1312.

88 Lionakis MS, Lewis RE, Torres HA, Albert ND, Raad II, Kontoyiannis DP: Increased frequency of non-fumigatus *Aspergillus* species in amphotericin B- or triazole-pre-exposed cancer patients with positive cultures for aspergilli. Diagn Microbiol Infect Dis 2005;52:15–20.

89 Herbrecht R, Denning DW, Patterson TF, Bennett JE, Greene RE, Oestmann JW, Kern WV, Marr KA, Ribaud P, Lortholary O, Sylvester R, Rubin RH, Wingard JR, Stark P, Durand C, Caillot D, Thiel E, Chandrasekar PH, Hodges MR, Schlamm HT, Troke PF, de Pauw B: Voriconazole versus amphotericin B for primary therapy of invasive aspergillosis. N Engl J Med 2002;347:408–415.

90 Imhof A, Balajee SA, Fredricks DN, Englund JA, Marr KA: Breakthrough fungal infections in stem cell transplant recipients receiving voriconazole. Clin Infect Dis 2004;39:743–746.

91 Marty FM, Cosimi LA, Baden LR: Breakthrough zygomycosis after voriconazole treatment in recipients of hematopoietic stem-cell transplants. N Engl J Med 2004;350:950–952.

92 Siwek GT, Dodgson KJ, de Magalhaes-Silverman M, Bartelt LA, Kilborn SB, Hoth PL, Diekema DJ, Pfaller MA: Invasive zygomycosis in hematopoietic stem cell transplant recipients receiving voriconazole prophylaxis. Clin Infect Dis 2004;39:584–587.

93 Mattner F, Weissbrodt H, Strueber M: Two case reports: fatal *Absidia corymbifera* pulmonary tract infection in the first postoperative phase of a lung transplant patient receiving voriconazole prophylaxis, and transient bronchial *Absidia corymbifera* colonization in a lung transplant patient. Scand J Infect Dis 2004;36:312–314.

94 Ifran A, Kaptan K, and Beyan C: Efficacy of caspofungin in prophylaxis and treatment of an adult leukemic patient with invasive pulmonary aspergillosis in allogeneic stem cell transplantation. Mycoses 2005;48:146–148.

95 Perfect JR: Management of invasive mycoses in hematology patients: current approaches. Oncology (Huntingt) 2004;18:5–14.

96 Perfect JR: Use of newer antifungal therapies in clinical practice: what do the data tell us? Oncology (Williston Park) 2004;18:15–23.

97 van Burik JA, Ratanatharathorn V, Stepan DE, Miller CB, Lipton JH, Vesole DH, Bunin N, Wall DA, Hiemenz JW, Satoi Y, Lee JM, Walsh TJ: Micafungin versus fluconazole for prophylaxis against invasive fungal infections during neutropenia in patients undergoing hematopoietic stem cell transplantation. Clin Infect Dis 2004;39:1407–1416.

98 Walsh TJ, Teppler H, Donowitz GR, Maertens JA, Baden LR, Dmoszynska A, Cornely OA, Bourque MR, Lupinacci RJ, Sable CA, dePauw BE: Caspofungin versus liposomal amphotericin B for empirical antifungal therapy in patients with persistent fever and neutropenia. N Engl J Med 2004;351:1391–1402.



Beth Arthington-Skaggs, PhD
Global AIDS Program, Centers for Disease Control and Prevention
JAT Complex, Building 4, 267 Av. Zedequias Manganhela, 7th Floor H1/H2
Maputo (Mozambique)
Tel. +258 84 304 5046, Fax +258 21 314 460, E-Mail skaggsb@mz.cdc.gov

Weber JT (ed): Antimicrobial Resistance – Beyond the Breakpoint.
Issues Infect Dis. Basel, Karger, 2010, vol 6, pp 154–170

# Preparing for HIV Drug Resistance in the Developing World

Diane E. Bennett

Global AIDS Program, Centers for Disease Control and Prevention, Atlanta, Ga., USA

## Abstract

HIV drug resistance (HIVDR) inevitably emerges with antiretroviral treatment (ART), because HIV has a high turnover rate and mutates easily, and because ART is lifelong. Inadequate drug pressure leads to quick evolution of resistant HIV. Currently only 42% of eligible individuals in resource-limited countries are receiving ART, but plans for quick ART scale-up are progressing. Their effectiveness could be jeopardized by drug resistance if HIVDR prevention is not incorporated into scale-up plans. ART programs in resource-limited countries are as successful as those in high-income countries. Challenges will come in maintaining high success rates as ART is expanded and decentralized. Most factors associated with treatment interruption and development of resistance are programmatic: costs to the patient associated with care, transport difficulties and interruptions in drug supplies. Optimal regimens and viral load testing to support HIVDR prevention are unavailable to many patients because of their high costs to national programs, and lack of infrastructure. WHO recommends an HIV drug resistance prevention and assessment strategy, emphasizing good ART program practices, continuous drug supplies, support for access and adherence, and planning based on ART program monitoring and drug resistance. If resource-limited countries receive sufficient support and develop an infrastructure for coordinated ART delivery and evidence-based HIVDR prevention, the threat to effective treatment posed by drug resistance can be controlled.



## HIV Drug Resistance and Antiretroviral Treatment Scale-Up in Resource-Limited Countries

In the early years of this century, some scientists feared that providing antiretroviral treatment (ART) to millions of HIV-infected individuals in resource-limited countries could lead to rapid emergence and transmission of drug-resistant HIV (DR-HIV), which could render ART ineffective [1, 2]. In 2001, Andrew Natsios, then administrator of the United States Agency for International Development, stated that the USA would emphasize aid for HIV prevention rather than HIV treatment. He said that treatment would be ineffective and drug resistance was likely to result from ART in Africa because Africans 'do not know what Western time is' and 'do not know what you are talking about' when asked to take drugs at specific times [3]. However, HIV-infected persons whose infections have progressed to AIDS are likely to die within 1 year; the imperative to save lives led to a commitment to ART for resource-limited countries [4]. Natsios's concerns about African adherence have proved unfounded, as studies have now shown that in sub-Saharan Africa adherence is often better than in high-income countries [5, 6].

A public health strategy was developed for ART to be extended rapidly to individuals in need [7] based on standardized simplified treatment protocols, standardized management approaches and decentralized service delivery. Clinicians do not make individualized ART decisions: ART start, determination of ART failure, and regimen selection is a matter of national policy guided by World Health Organization (WHO) recommendations [8]. This approach enables health-care workers with minimum training to deliver care to large numbers of patients in facilities without sophisticated resources.

The basis of ART scale-up is 1 potent first-line regimen and 1 alternate, both consisting of 1 non-nucleoside reverse transcriptase inhibitor (NNRTI) supported by 2 nucleoside/nucleotide reverse transcriptase inhibitors (NRTIs), and 1 second-line regimen, based on 2 NRTIs and a protease inhibitor (PI) such as lopinavir whose efficacy is 'boosted' (enhanced) by another PI, ritonavir, in low doses. National selection of the first-line regimen for the population takes into account as far as possible efficacy, durability and tolerability (the criteria used in high-income countries), but also whether the ARVs are registered and marketed in the country, especially in fixed-dose combinations [9], their cost [10, 11] and whether drugs can be transported and stored unrefrigerated [10]. Second-line regimens for each country are based on WHO recommendations but in-country selection is based on primarily on availability and affordability of a regimen and, to the extent possible, its ability to minimize the effect of cross-resistance after a first-line failure [12]. Given limited laboratory facilities, decisions to start, substitute one first-line ARV for another, or switch to second-line treatment are generally made on the basis of clinical observation and WHO clinical staging or, if available, CD4 count [13], hemotology and biochemistry. In some sites in African and Asian countries, the decision to switch to second-line treatment is also based on viral load. Viral load measurements are now recommended by WHO for determination of ART failure [6], but they are unlikely to be routinely performed in all sites in many resource-limited countries due to cost, complexity and lack of laboratory facilities.

National ART policy is based on WHO guidelines in almost all countries where ART scale-up is taking place [13, 14]. The rapid scale-up of ART for HIV in resource-limited countries has become an international priority, although recent economic difficulties may slow the pace of expansion. The G8 countries and the United Nations member states have endorsed the global goal of universal access to ART by 2010, and the WHO, the Joint United Nations Program on AIDS (UNAIDS), the US President's Emergency Plan for AIDS Relief, the Global Fund to Fight AIDS, Tuberculosis, and Malaria, and numerous countries and partner organizations are heavily committed to supporting ART expansion. At the end of 2008, it was estimated that more than 4 million people were receiving ART in low- and middle-income countries, representing coverage of 42% of the estimated 9.5 million people in need of ART [15]. The 2 areas where over 90% of individuals in need of ART reside are sub-Saharan Africa and South/South-East Asia. As of December 2008, sub-Saharan Africa was estimated to have more than 2.9 million people on ART, with coverage of 44% of the 6.7 million in need, whereas in 2003 there were 100,000 on treatment and coverage was only 2%. In East, South and South-East Asia, 656,000 people (37% of the 1.5 million in need) were receiving ART in December 2008, a 9-fold increase compared with the 70,000 receiving ART at the end of 2003. Expansion has been rapid, but the need remains great. Most countries have targeted coverage for 80% of individuals in need of ART as their 2010 goal [16]. How likely is it that drug resistant HIV will render ART ineffective as the scale-up is taking place?

*Development of Drug-Resistant Strains of HIV*

Generalizing from other organisms, journalists often imagine that emerging HIV drug resistance will take the form of one or more super-strains of multi-drug-resistant HIV that will quickly spread across countries and continents, but in fact the evolution and widespread transmission of 1 powerful strain of multi-resistant HIV is unlikely. Resistant strains of HIV are on the whole less fit than drug-sensitive strains, and most are less transmissible (and HIV itself is far less transmissible than most infectious organisms). No individual resistant strain has ever been identified among a large number of individuals; only 1 chain of transmission in more than 20 people has been reported in scientific literature, with the report demonstrating transmission over 3 years among 24 individuals of an NNRTI-resistant strain in a network with a high rate of partner change [17]. Resistance patterns that are common among individuals do not generally result from their being infected with a common strain of HIV.

The viral dynamics of HIV provide an explanation for this phenomenon. Resistance to ARVs occurs because of mutations that emerge in the HIV genetic material coding for proteins whose functioning is targeted by ARVs. Specific mutations make the proteins less vulnerable to the drugs that target them, and during replication HIV is prone to mutations [18]. Coupled with its high mutation rate, the high level of virus in infected individuals and the rapid rate of viral turnover [19] ensure an infected individual actually has a multitude of slightly different strains of HIV ('quasi-species'). Most mutations create new HIV strains that cannot survive or replicate, but some of the new strains are viable. When an individual takes a non-potent or intermittent ARV regimen, strains with mutations that are resistant to one or more drugs in the regimen will evolve and quickly multiply to become the predominant circulating strains of HIV within the individual. Emergence of any one strain of resistant HIV as predominant within an infected individual depends on the interaction between the concentrations of ARV drugs in the various compartments of the body, the current population of HIV quasi-species within the individual, and the individual's own immune system.

Fortunately, resistance-related mutations generally make HIV less fit than 'wild-type' (drug sensitive) HIV in the absence of drug pressure [20], so that resistant strains that arise spontaneously do not become the predominant viral population in an untreated individual. Also, when a potent ARV regimen produces suppression of HIV below measurable levels, viral evolution and replication are suppressed to a level where new resistant strains that arise do not replicate or remain in memory cells. To minimize the risk of development and replication of strains with new resistance mutations, ART should ideally maintain plasma HIV-1 RNA levels below the limits of detection of the commercially available assays (<50–400 copies/ml) [21].

*Classes of Antiretroviral Drugs and Treatment Strategies in Resource-Limited Countries*

Three major classes of ARVs are in common use, all of which target enzymes (proteins) that are crucial to HIV's life cycle. NRTIs act as DNA chain terminators and inhibit reverse transcription of the viral RNA genome into DNA, preventing a key early stage in HIV's lifecycle; NNRTIs bind and prevent the action of reverse transcriptase, and PIs prevent the enzyme protease from cleaving precursor proteins from which the inner core of viral particles is assembled [22]. Only these 3 ARV classes are likely to be used to any great extent in resource-limited countries according to current plans, because these drugs are potent, easy to manage and well-tolerated, relatively cheap, often available as fixed-dose combinations. In addition, newer drug classes are extremely expensive, require more complex management and have not been registered by manufacturers for use in many developing countries. Standard regimens consist of 3 or more drugs from at least 2 different classes, used in combination to inhibit viral replication at multiple steps of the replication cycle. With all ART, drug pressure can be sub-optimal if treatment is interrupted, a non-potent regimen has been prescribed, or if ARV drug concentrations within the body are insufficient due to interactions with other drugs or the individual's own metabolism. In the presence of sub-optimal drug levels, an DR-HIV strain can evolve and become the predominant circulating strain within an individual after only 2–4 weeks [23].

Mutations contributing to resistance to these 3 major drug classes develop in the regions of the HIV *pol* gene that code for the protease or reverse transcriptase enzymes. Different mutations confer or support resistance to different antiretroviral drugs or drug classes, and a particular resistance pattern may require a longer duration of inadequate drug pressure to develop. Each position in the HIV genome has 3 nucleotides that code for 1 amino acid in the relevant enzyme. If the predominant wild-type nucleotide triplet must undergo only 1 change to create the amino acid associated with resistance, the 'genetic barrier' to resistance is said to be low; if it requires 2 or more changes, the genetic barrier is higher. The genetic barrier is also based on the number of nucleotide mutations at different positions needed to confer resistance. PI resistance has a high genetic barrier with many mutations generally required and the NNRTIs have a low genetic barrier, requiring as little as 1 nucleotide change in 1 mutation.

In contrast to the natural history of drug-resistant strains that develop in many other organisms, a DR-HIV subpopulation that achieves predominance in an individual under inadequate drug pressure will generally not remain predominant in the circulation when the incomplete drug pressure is removed. Commonly transmitted drug-sensitive wild-type HIV has evolved to be more 'fit' and to have a higher capacity to replicate within the human body in the absence of drug pressure than resistant strains [20]. If drug pressure ceases, wild-type HIV will outgrow the drug resistant strains quickly, again within 2 weeks to 1 month, and will become the predominant circulating strain once again. After stopping ART, the individual is unlikely to transmit drug-resistant HIV after a few weeks to months. However, previously acquired drug-resistant strains remain present within memory cells and will quickly replicate and become predominant again in an individual patient if the same drugs are restarted. Most drug-resistant strains are not resistant to all drugs and all drug classes, so after treatment failure suppression by a potent regimen to which these strains are not resistant is generally possible if the new regimen includes a new drug class [21]. If the new regimen is successful, replication of strains resistant to the previous regimen are effectively suppressed along with drug-sensitive strains. Also, residual anti-HIV activity remains even after development of resistance to NRTIs and boosted PIs [21], viral loads are substantially lower and some clinical benefit remains if ART with a regimen to which resistance has developed is maintained, and patients do substantially worse if ART is stopped. Maintaining a patient on a regimen to which resistance has developed is recommended if no alternative regimens are available.

To prevent viral replication and maximize quality of life for an individual in treatment, HIV replication should be effectively suppressed for the longest possible period of time with the initial regimen. NNRTI-based first-line regimens have fewer side effects and are cheaper than PI-based regimens, hence the recommendation for their use in first-line regimens in resource-limited countries. If the first regimen fails, a second regimen should be instituted to which drug-resistant strains evolved under the first regimen are likely to be sensitive, and so on. Prevention of DR-HIV depends on viral suppression and the use of appropriate regimens both initially and following treatment failure. Use of a single drug initially generates resistant strains fairly quickly, and the addition of a single new drug to a failing regimen generally leads to generation of resistance mutations and subsequent failure.


*Factors Potentially Associated with HIV Drug Resistance in Resource-Limited Countries*


Many aspects of the public health ART strategy, where it is successfully implemented, support limitation of DR-HIV. Except in the few countries like India with a substantial private sector where inappropriate prescribing may be a problem, nearly all ART patients are treated with potent 3-drug regimens that can reliably suppress HIV replication to levels <50 copies/ml, also suppressing the emergence and replication of drug-resistant strains. The availability of a limited number of regimens limits unnecessary switching; the use of fixed dose combinations supports adherence [24] and limits selective drug-taking [25]. Widespread prescribing of inappropriate ART is seen more frequently in countries where many different ARV drugs are available, such as Mexico [26], than in countries following the public health approach with a limited number of regimens used in the public sector.

Despite earlier doubts, evidence is available that even in countries with very limited resources, ART programs based on the public health approach have shown effectiveness equal to that seen in clinical cohorts in the USA and Europe using similar regimens [27–33]. A major challenge is to replicate these optimal outcomes in new ART sites as ART is expanded to approach universal access. Training additional personnel, and retaining currently trained staff when more lucrative jobs may be offered in high-income countries or when they themselves may be HIV-infected [34], and expansion of supervision, monitoring, laboratory services and drug delivery systems are major challenges. In this context there are many potential sources of interruptions to treatment, or suboptimal treatment, which can lead to insufficient drug pressure and DR-HIV.

Patient adherence in resource-limited countries has been reported as higher than in high-income countries [6, 35, 36], though many of the studies are small. The individual factors facilitating non-adherence and resulting treatment interruptions are similar to those in high-income countries [37]. Fixed-dose combinations, fewer pills and less frequent dosing facilitate adherence. However, programmatic barriers to continuous ART access play a greater role in non-continuous drug taking and preventable DR-HIV emergence in resource-limited countries. Barriers include charges for treatment or drugs [28, 38–42] as well as long distances to be traveled to ART sites and lack of affordable transport [1, 43, 44]. Interruption of ARV supplies at both site and country level also leads to ART interruptions [45–47]; ongoing efforts are required to support drug supply continuity. Failure to pick up drugs on time may result from transport difficulties, illness, other obligations or lack of funds where payment is required. Even if drugs are picked as few as 48 h after previously dispensed drugs run out, the interruption may result in NNRTI resistance [48] because an NNRTI will persist at subtherapeutic levels in the human body longer than NRTIs, leading to the equivalent of monotherapy. Failure to pick up ARV drugs before drugs picked up previously would have run out has been shown in numerous studies to be a major predictor of viral failure and the development of resistance [45, 49]. Temporary 'losses to follow-up' from ART programs or ART stops may also be sources of resistance [45, 50, 51]. Particularly if adherence was less than perfect beforehand, a lapse in clinic attendance of days to months may lead to NNRTI resistance. If the patient eventually returns for ART, he or she is likely in most resource-limited countries to be re-started on the same first-line regimen, to which there may be archived NNRTI resistance. These sources of drug resistance are to some extent preventable by the application of targeted resources within the existing public health approach in existing programs [52, 53]. Maintaining continuity of treatment during human conflict and natural disasters is especially challenging, though careful planning and targeting of resources have minimized interruptions in some settings [54].

Some aspects of the public health approach as currently implemented could be associated with the emergence of additional resistance mutations during failing ART regimens. The most common first-line regimens in countries following the public health approach currently consist of stavudine (d4T) or zidovudine (AZT) plus lamivudine and an NNRTI [55]. Although new WHO guidelines recommend phasing out d4T due to its relative toxicity [6], its very low cost and efficacy may mean that some countries will continue its use. Because toxicity is associated with reduced adherence, this could contribute to drug resistance. Clinical or immunological determinations of ART failure in the absence of viral load monitoring are associated with unnecessary switches to second-line ART in the absence of virological failure, but also with the prolongation of a failing regimen and a later switch to second line [56–58]. Later switches for a failing first-line regimen that includes NRTIs are associated with the accumulation of thymidine analogue and other resistance mutations [57, 59, 60], which can cause cross-resistance to many – and possibly all – NRTIs that might be used in a second-line regimen. This phenomenon has been reported among many failures in some countries [61], and more rarely in others [62]. It may be less likely when tenofovir (TDF) is included in the first-line regimen [63], but TDF availability is still limited in resource-limited countries and it is substantially more expensive than other NRTIs [9]. Even with viral load testing available, the patterns of resistance developed may severely limit NRTI options for second-line regimens [12]. There is some evidence that second-line ART regimens combining a boosted PI with NRTIs may be sufficiently potent to succeed despite the presence of NRTI mutations [64]. A greater problem is the absence of second-line availability: key drugs in WHO-recommended second-line regimens, including TDF, abacavir (ABC), and ritonavir-boosted PIs are still limited or unaffordable in many countries, although prices have decreased substantially [9, 65]. Changing a patient's regimen from first-line to second-line raises the cost between 9-fold in countries where generic drugs are available to 17-fold in middle-income countries where patent protections are in force [9].

There is little chance that salvage ART regimens (to be used after a second-line regimen has failed) including new drug classes will be widely available in resource-limited countries during the next 5 years, because of their cost and complexity and because there is little economic incentive for pharmaceutical companies to register them in resource-limited countries. Companies may not make drugs available at affordable prices even if they are registered in countries. Although competition among generic manufacturers has reduced the price of first generation of ARVs more than 99% since the year 2000, new patenting regulations make it unlikely that the newer drug classes will benefit from a similar phenomenon. The World Trade Organization's Trade-Related Aspect of Intellectual Property Rights agreement, honored by 148 countries, requires pharmaceutical patents for the newer drug classes. All resource-limited countries were required to provide patent protection for new pharmaceutical products as of 2005. India, which produces 90% of the ARVs used in resource-limited countries, initiated patent laws then. Because relatively few individuals are taking second-line regimens currently, the lack of salvage regimens is unlikely to contribute substantially to resistance at this time. However, eventually the necessity of maintaining patients on a failing second-line regimen may also contribute to the emergence of resistance. In resource-limited countries, successfully treating patients for as long as possible on uninterrupted first-line ART, which is simpler to administer, associated with higher levels of adherence, and less costly than second-line ART, is crucial to both prevention of resistance and supporting good health for individuals living with HIV [53]. Reports have shown that adverse events (toxicity) during a first-line regimens may sometimes trigger unnecessary switches to more complex second-line regimens where appropriate alternate first-line ARVs for substitution are unavailable because of cost [66].

## HIV Drug Resistance Associated with Prevention of Mother-to-Child HIV Transmission

NNRTI resistance mutations have been reported in 20–69% of women [67–69] who have received single-dose nevirapine (sd-NVP) to prevent HIV transmission to a child during pregnancy. However, although suboptimal with regard to resistance, for programmatic reasons sd-NVP is the most common ARV prophylaxis intervention used for prevention of mother-to-child transmission (PMTCT) of HIV in resource-limited countries because of its safety, efficacy, simplicity and low cost [70, 71]. NNRTI mutations associated with sd-NVP, unlike those that appear with inadequate ART-associated drug pressure lasting weeks to months, are reported not to affect the outcome of ART provided it commences more than 6–12 months after PMTCT [72]. The short duration of sd-NVP exposure may limit the number of DR-HIV strains in memory cells [73]. An increasing number of eligible women are receiving PMTCT in resource-limited countries (45% worldwide and 58% in Eastern and Southern Africa as of December 2008 [1, 15]), and mutations associated with sd-NVP may have an adverse effect on those who receive ART for less than 6 months. Increasingly, women eligible for ART during pregnancy are receiving potent 3-drug ART [74]. For those not ART eligible, PMTCT utilizing ARV combinations to minimize resistance is recommended [75], and its provision is increasing in many countries, though greater complexity of administration and cost may limit expansion of this option. New recommendations for prolongation of PMTCT during pregnancy and to cover the period of breast feeding [75] may have a mixed effect on the emergence of DR-HIV. Longer duration of PMTCT will prevent

HIV transmission more effectively, but also produces more opportunities for poor adherence, which could result in transmission of resistant strains.

NNRTI resistance is widespread in HIV-infected infants whose mothers have received NVP monotherapy for PMTCT or who themselves receive NVP monotherapy. This resistance has been associated with failure of NNRTI-based regimens subsequently used for pediatric ART [68]. However, because 85–95% of infants whose mothers or who themselves receive NPV monotherapy do not become HIV-infected [76], this is currently a relatively infrequent cause of resistance in children on a population basis. However, direct administration to infants of NVP for PMTCT is also increasing (35% in 2008), and is another potential source of resistance in children that could affect NNRTI-based ART adversely. In April 2008, WHO revised its pediatric ARV guidelines [77] to recommend the use of the boosted PI lopinavir/ritonavir (LPV/r) for infants who have been exposed to an NNRTI either directly or through their mothers. This recommendation is scientifically justified, but LPV/r syrup for children is 70% more expensive than a liquid NNRTI-based regimen, and requires refrigeration, and for both reasons may not be widely used in resource-limited countries [77]. Development of pediatric versions of heat-stable PIs should be prioritized.

Treatment failure and DR-HIV emergence in children in resource-limited countries is also associated with inappropriate use of adult formulations because pediatric formulations are unavailable, because doses do not take into account changes in weight, and because of adherence problems [77]. Finally, there are several available pediatric fixed-dose combination ARVs that come in doses for various child sizes, but of the 22 ARVs approved by the US Food and Drug Administration for adults, 6 are not approved for use in children and 7 have no pediatric formulations [78]. Most pediatric formulations are not yet well adapted for use in resource-limited settings: they come in powder or syrup forms and many need to be mixed with clean water or require refrigeration. Even after this problem has been solved, strategies to address access barriers and adherence support will be urgently needed.


**Transmission of HIV Drug Resistance**

The prevalence of transmitted HIV drug resistance depends on many factors, but one of the most important is ART use, that is, the extent to which ART is used in an area, how long it has been widely used, and the numbers and percentages of those who are currently on a failing regimen [79–81]. In most resource-limited countries, 15–20% of HIV-infected individuals are estimated to be in need of ART [15], and only 45% of these received ART in 2008; in 2003, only 2% of those in need were receiving ART [15]. Based on these figures, models predict transmitted HIV drug resistance at a level of ≥5% is unlikely for many years in most of these countries [79–81]. Because the majority of ART patients are starting on highly potent regimens [7], the rise of drug resistance transmission is likely to be delayed compared to high-income countries, where ART scale-up was initially implemented with resistance-associated monotherapy and 1-class dual therapy. The effect of maintaining individuals on a failing regimen in the absence of viral load testing may contribute to transmitted drug resistance as the duration of widespread ART increases in countries, although the extent of this contribution requires more study. Residual ARV activity and partial viral suppression is often seen in individuals taking a regimen to which resistance has developed [82–84], which could lower the risk of transmission. Those who stop taking their drugs will not continue to transmit DR-HIV because the more fit drug-sensitive strains will quickly take over as majority quasi-species in the absence of drug pressure. Also, the proportion of patients not eligible for ART, plus those who are eligible but are not receiving ART, will continue to be much higher than the proportion receiving ART; transmission risks are likely to be congruent with these proportions. Success in limiting risk behavior among ART patients can also decrease transmission of resistant strains. 'Prevention for positives' programs that focus on reducing risky behavior among patients in care, as well as supporting adherence, have demonstrated beneficial reduction in risk behaviors among ART patients in resource-limited countries, lowering the risk for HIV transmission, including transmission of resistant strains [85–88].

One potentially worrying finding is that drug-resistance mutations persist for much longer in the circulation among individuals whose resistant strains are due to transmission rather than acquired during treatment [89, 90]. In high-income countries, transmission chains from individuals who themselves have a primary infection with DR-HIV has been well-documented [17, 91]. Fortunately, such chains of transmission are reported among relatively few individuals in high-income countries where transmitted resistance levels are much higher than in resource-limited countries, and as previously stated, the relative proportions of newly infected individuals with transmitted DR-HIV are likely to remain low in resource-limited countries for many years.

WHO recommends a public health approach to surveillance and prevention of resistance rather than a strategy based on laboratory testing for resistance in individual patients [92]. This strategy is integrated into the national HIV treatment and care plan. The most important drug resistance assessment does not involve laboratory testing. HIV drug resistance 'early warning indicators' (ART program factors known to be associated with drug resistance and susceptible to preventive action) are abstracted from medical and pharmacy records in all ART sites in a country, or a large number of representative sites, and public health action is taken to improve site functioning [92]. These include: prescribing practices; losses to follow-up; the extent to which patients are still on an appropriate first-line ART regimen 12 months after starting ART; the extent to which patients pick up ARV drugs before previous drugs would have run out; clinic appointment keeping, and continuity of ARV drug supplies. Site profiles are collected annually on costs of care to patients, clinic and pharmacy hours, distances and costs of transport, type and extent of adherence support and support for follow-up of patients who do not return. Many countries report sites have insufficient resources to ensure adequate follow-up for patients who do not return and to support patients in picking up their ARV drugs on time, particularly where transport costs are a problem. Other countries report that lack of drug supply continuity at ART sites is a major problem. Charges for laboratory tests and other clinical services (not generally for ARV drugs) are a continuing barrier to continuity of care, particularly in some Asian countries.

WHO also recommends that countries conduct limited laboratory surveys in sentinel ART sites to evaluate baseline resistance in patients starting ART, and factors associated with virologic failure and resistance 12 months after ART start [93]. The third assessment element consists of small surveys to assess transmitted DR-HIV in capital cities and other areas where ART has been widespread for at least 3 years [94, 95]. So far, surveys from 11 resource-limited countries have demonstrated no substantial transmission of DR-HIV [95, 96]. DR-HIV prevention elements recommended by WHO include support for adherence and follow-up, minimizing barriers to continuous access to care, training clinical staff about appropriate prescribing and care, and focused efforts to enhance drug supply continuity at the country, provincial and site level.

Substantial progress has been made in providing life-saving ART in resource-limited countries, and in implementing measures which will limit the emergence and transmission of drug resistance. Costs of many ARV drugs have been lowered substantially [9], and more fixed-dose combinations, which foster adherence [97], are available [9]. The recent 'patent pool' for ARV drugs put in place by UNITAID could further reduce costs [98]. Drug supply systems have improved in many countries, but treatment interruptions due to supply shortages continue to be widely reported [78]. Decentralization to smaller ART sites will not only make treatment available to more patients, but will cut-down travel time and transport costs which contribute to ART interruption. On the other hand, substantial stigma [99–103] is still attached to HIV infection, causing many patients to continue to choose clinics far away from their homes for treatment or to miss picking up their drugs on time. A lack of essential laboratory tests to monitor adverse reactions (which contribute to ART interruptions) and to determine ART failure causes substantial difficulty in many countries; adverse reactions, as well as contributing to morbidity, are associated with reduced adherence and drug resistance [65, 104, 105]. Development of low-cost, feasible laboratory tests and laboratory infrastructure to support optimal HIV care should be prioritized.


**Summary**

HIV drug resistance is associated with ART in all countries of the world. ART programs in resource-limited countries demonstrate equal success in preventing treatment failure compared with programs in centers of excellence in high-income countries. There is little evidence that patients in resource-limited countries are less capable of ART adherence than those in high-income countries, and some evidence that they do better.

                                                          Bennett

Most of the problems contributing to drug resistance in resource-limited countries are preventable: continuity of drug supplies must be maintained through better planning and delivery systems, and barriers to access to care such as transport and treatment costs, lack of resources for adherence support and follow-up of non-returning patients, and inconvenient clinic and pharmacy hours, should be addressed. Better pediatric formulations, better PMTCT regimens, and implementation of viral load testing are crucial, and cheaper fixed dose combinations, including those for treatment after initial regimens have failed, should be developed and made available for both adults and children. Meeting the urgent need to continue scaling up ART is challenging, given the minimal health infrastructure, lack of trained personnel and facilities, complexities of drug ordering, delivery and storage, and inadequate laboratory capacity in many resource-limited countries. Renewed international commitment will be required to address the needs of these countries and their ART programs.

## References


1 Stevens W, Kaye S, Corrah T: Antiviral therapy in Africa. BMJ 2004;328:260–262.

2 Harries AD, Nyangulu DS, Hargreaves NJ, Kaluwa O, Salaniponi FM: Preventing antiretroviral anarchy in sub-Saharan Africa. Lancet 2001;358:1819–1820.

3 Boston Globe, June 7, 2001, p A8.

4 Moatti JP, Spire B, and Kazatchkine M: Drug resistance and adherence to HIV/AIDS antiretroviral treatment: against a double standard between the north and the south. AIDS 2004;18(suppl 3):S55–S61.

5 Crane JT, Kawuma A, Oyugi JH, Byakika JT, Moss A, Bourgois P, Bangsberg DR: The price of adherence: qualitative findings from HIV positive individuals purchasing fixed-dose combination generic HIV antiretroviral therapy in Kampala, Uganda. AIDS Behav 2006;10:437–442.

6 Ware NC, Idoko J, Kaaya S, Biraro IA, Wyatt MA, Agbaji O, Chalamilla G, Bangsberg DR: Explaining adherence success in sub-Saharan Africa: an ethnographic study. PLoS Med 2009;6:e11.

7 Gilks CF, Crowley S, Ekpini R, Gove S, Perriens J, Souteyrand Y, Sutherland D, Vitoria M, Guerman T, De Cock K: The WHO public-health approach to antiretroviral treatment against HIV in resource-limited settings. Lancet 2006;368:505–510.

8 World Health Organization. Rapid Advice: Antiviral Therapy for HIV Infection in Adults and Adolescents. 2009 World Health Organization, Geneva, Switzerland. (Accessed December 24, 2009).

9 Médecins Sans Frontières: Untangling the web of price reductions: a pricing guide for the purchase of ARVs for developing countries, ed 11. 2008. www.accessmed-msf.org/fileadmin/user_upload/diseases/hiv-aids/Untangling_the_Web/Untanglingtheweb_July2008_English.pdf (accessed December 15, 2009).

10 Ford N, Wilson D, Costa CG, Lotrowska M, Kijtiwatchakul K: Sustaining access to antiretroviral therapy in the less-developed world: lessons from Brazil and Thailand. AIDS, 2007;21(suppl 4):S21–S29.

11 Pinheiroa E, Wasanb A, Kimb JY, Leed E, Guimierd, JM, and Perriens J. Examining the production costs of antiretroviral drugs. AIDS 2006;20:1745–1752.

12 Sungkanuparph,S, Manosuthi W, Kiertiburanakul S, et al: Options for a second-line antiretroviral regimen for HIV type 1-infected patients whose initial regimen of a fixed-dose combination of stavudine, lamivudine, and nevirapine fails. Clin Infect Dis 2007;44:447–452.

13 World Health Organization: WHO case definitions of HIV for surveillance and revised clinical staging and immunological classification of HIV-related disease in adults and children. 2007. www.who.int/hiv/pub/guidelines/HIVstaging150307.pdf (accessed May 1, 2009).

14 Beck EJ, Vitoria M, Mandalia S, Crowley S, Gilks CF, Souteyrand Y: National adult antiretroviral therapy guidelines in resource-limited countries: concordance with 2003 WHO guidelines? AIDS 2006;20:1497–1502.

15  World Health Organization; Joint United Nations Programme on HIV/AIDS; UNICEF: Towards universal access: scaling up priority HIV/AIDS interventions in the health sector. Progress report 2009. www.who.int/hiv/pub/towards_universal_access_report_2009.pdf (accessed January 2, 2010).

16  Joint United Nations Programme on HIV/AIDS: Financial resources required to achieve universal access to hiv prevention, treatment, care and support. 2007. http://data.unaids.org/pub/Report/2007/2007 0925_advocacy_grne2_en.pdf (accessed October 1, 2008).

17  Brenner BG, Roger M, Moisi DD, Oliveira M, Hardy I, Turgel R, Charest H, Routy JP, Wainberg MA: Transmission networks of drug resistance acquired in primary/early stage HIV infection. AIDS 2008; 22:2509–2515.

18  Coffin JM: HIV population dynamics in vivo: implications for genetic variation, pathogenesis, and therapy. Science 1995;267:483–489.

19  Perelson AS, Neumann AU, Markowitz M, Leonard JM, Ho DD: HIV-1 dynamics in vivo: virion clearance rate, infected cell life-span, and viral generation time. Science 1996;271:1582–1586.

20  Bangsberg DR, Acosta EP, Gupta R, Guzman D, Riley ED, Harrigan PR, Parkin N, Deeks SG: Adherence-resistance relationships for protease and non-nucleoside reverse transcriptase inhibitors explained by virological fitness. AIDS 2006;20:223–231.

21  Hammer SM, Eron JJ Jr, Reiss P, Schooley RT, Thompson MA, Walmsley S, Cahn P, Fischl MA, Gatell JM, Hirsch MS, Jacobsen DM, Montaner JS, Richman DD, Yeni PG, Volberding PA: Antiretroviral treatment of adult HIV infection: 2008 recommendations of the International AIDS Society-USA panel. JAMA 2008;300:555–570.

22  Clavel F, Race E, Mammano F: HIV drug resistance and viral fitness. Adv Pharmacol 2000;49:41–66.

23  Wei X, Ghosh S, Taylor ME, Johnson VA, Emini EA, Deutsch P, Lifson JD, Bonhoeffer S, Nowak MA, Hahn BH, Saag MS, Shaw GM: Viral dynamics in human immunodeficiency virus type 1 infection. Nature 1995;373:117–122.

24  Crane JT, Kawuma A, Oyugi JH, Byakika JT, Moss A, Bourgois P, Bangsberg DR: The price of adherence: qualitative findings from HIV positive individuals purchasing fixed-dose combination generic HIV antiretroviral therapy in Kampala, Uganda. AIDS Behav 2006;10:437–442.

25  Gardner EM, Burman WJ, Maravi ME, Davidson AJ: Selective drug taking during combination antiretroviral therapy in an unselected clinic population. J Acquir Immune Defic Syndr 2005;40:294–300.

26  Bautista-Arredondo S, Mane A, Bertozzi SM: Economic impact of antiretroviral therapy prescription decisions in the context of rapid scaling-up of access to treatment: lessons from Mexico. AIDS 2006;20:101–109.

27  Garrido C, Zahonero N, Fernandes D, Serrano D, Silva AR, Ferraria N, Antunes F, Gonzalez-Lahoz J, Soriano V, de Mendoza C: Subtype variability, virological response and drug resistance assessed on dried blood spots collected from HIV patients on antiretroviral therapy in Angola. J Antimicrob Chemother 2008;61:694–698.

28  Ivers LC, Kendrick D, Doucette K: Efficacy of antiretroviral therapy programs in resource-poor settings: a meta-analysis of the published literature. Clinical Infectious Diseases 2005;41:217–224.

29  Severe P, Leger P, Charles M, Noel F, Bonhomme G, Bois B, George E, Kenel-Pierre S, Wright PF, Gulick R, Johnson WD, Pape JW, Fitzgerald DW: Antiretroviral therapy in a thousand patients with AIDS in Haiti. N Engl J Med 2006;353:2325–2331.

30  Ferradini L, Jeannin A, Pinoges L, Izopet J, Odhiambo D, Mankhambo L, Karungi G, Szumilin E, Balandine S, Fedida G, Carrieri MP, Spire B, Ford N, Tassie J-M, Guerin PJ, Brasher C: Scaling up of highly active antiretroviral therapy in a rural district of Malawi: an effectiveness assessment. Lancet 2006;367:1335–1342.

31  Sow PS, Otieno LF, Bissagnene E, Kityo C, Bennink R, Clevenbergh P, Wit FW, Waalberg E, Rinke de Wit TF, Lange JM: Implementation of an antiretroviral access program for HIV-1-infected individuals in resource-limited settings: clinical results from 4 African countries. J Acquir Immune Defic Syndr 2007;44:262–267.

32  Wools-Kaloustian K, Kimaiyo S, Diero L, Siika A, Sidle J, Yiannoutsos CT, Musick B, Einterz R, Fife KH, Tierney WM: Viability and effectiveness of large-scale HIV treatment initiatives in sub-Saharan Africa: experience from western Kenya. AIDS 2006; 20:41–48.

33  Keiser O, Orrell C, Egger M, Wood R, Brinkhof MW, Furrer H, Van Cutsem G, Ledergerber B, Boulle A: Public-health and individual approaches to antiretroviral therapy: township South Africa and Switzerland compared. PLoS Med 2008;5:e148.

34  Kinoti S, Tawfik L: The Impact of HIV/AIDS on the health workforce in developing countries: background paper prepared for the World Health Organization World Health Report. 2006.

35  Orrell C: Antiretroviral adherence in a resource-poor setting. Curr HIV/AIDS Rep 2005;2:171–176.

36 Oyugi JH, Byakika-Tusiime J, Charlebois ED, Kityo C, Mugerwa R, Mugyenyi P, Bangsberg DR: Multiple validated measures of adherence indicate high levels of adherence to generic HIV antiretroviral therapy in a resource-limited setting. J Acquir Immune Defic Syndr 2004;36:1100–1102.

37 Mills EJ, Nachega JB, Buchan I, Orbinski J, Attaran A, Singh S, Rachlis B, Wu P, Cooper C, Thabane L, Wilson K, Guyatt GH, Bangsberg DR: Adherence to antiretroviral therapy in Sub-Saharan Africa and North America: a meta-analysis. JAMA 2006;296:679–690.

38 Kabugo C, Bahendeka S, Mwebaze R, Malamba S, Katuntu D, Downing R, Mermin J, Weidle PJ: Long-term experience providing antiretroviral drugs in a fee-for-service HIV clinic in Uganda: evidence of extended virologic and CD4+ cell count responses. J Acquir Immune Defic Syndr 2005;38:578–583.

39 Colebunders R, Kamya M, Semitala F, Castelvuovo B, Katabira E, McAdam K: Free antiretrovirals must not be restricted only to treatment-naive patients. PLoS Med 2005;2:941–943.

40 Spacek LA, Shihab HM, Kamya MR, Mwesigire D, Ronald A, Mayanja H, Moore RD, Bates M, Quinn TC: Response to antiretroviral therapy in HIV-infected patients attending a public, urban clinic in Kampala, Uganda. Clin Infect Dis 2006;42:252–259.

41 Bisson GP, Frank I, Gross R, Lo Re V, Strom JB, Wanga X, Mogorosi M, Gaolathe T, Ndwapi N, Friednman H, Stroma BL, Dickinson D: Out-of-pocket costs of HAART limit HIV treatment responses in Botswana's private sector. AIDS 2006;20:1333–1336.

42 Weiser S, Wolfe W, Bangsberg D, Thior I, Gilbert P, Makhema J, Kebaabetswe P, Dickenson D, Mompati K, Essex M, Marlink R: Barriers to antiretroviral adherence for patients living with HIV Infection and AIDS in Botswana. J Acquir Immune Defic Syndr 2003;34:281–288.

43 Mukherjee JS, Ivers L, Leandre F: Antiretorivral Therapy in resource-poor settings: decreasing barriers to access and promoting adherence. J Acquir Immune Defic Syndr 2006;43:S123–S126.

44 Tuller DM, Bangsberg DR, Senkungu J, Ware NC, Emenyonu N, Weiser SD: Transportation costs impede sustained adherence and access to HAART in a clinic population in southwestern Uganda: a qualitative study. AIDS Behav 2009.

45 Oyugi JH, Byakika-Tusiime J, Ragland K, Laeyendecker O, Mugerwa R, Kityo C, Mugyenyi P, Quinn TC, Bangsberg DR: Treatment interruptions predict resistance in HIV-positive individuals purchasing fixed-dose combination antiretroviral therapy in Kampala, Uganda. AIDS 2007;21:965–971.

46 Okeke IN, Klugman KP, Bhutta ZA, Duse AG, Jenkins P, O'Brien TF, Pablos-Mendex A, Laxminarayan R: Antimicrobial resistance in developing countries. Part II. Strategies for containment. Lancet Infect Dis 2005;5:568–580.

47 Laurent C, Meilo H, Guiard-Schmid JB, Mapoure Y, Noël JM, M'Bangué M: Antiretroviral therapy in public and private routine health care clinics in Cameroon: lessons from the Douala antiretroviral (DARVIR) initiative. Clin Infect Dis 2005;41:108–111.

48 Gardner EM, Burman WJ, Steiner JF, Anderson PL, Bangsberg DR: Antiretroviral medication adherence and the development of class-specific antiretroviral resistance. AIDS 2009;23:1035–1046.

49 Bisson GP, Gross R, Bellamy S, Chittams J, Hislop M, Regensberg L, Frank I, Maartens G, Nachega JB: Pharmacy refill adherence compared with CD4 count changes for monitoring HIV-infected adults on antiretroviral therapy. PLoS Med 2008;5:e109.

50 Kamya MR, Mayanja-Kizza H, Kambugu A, Bakeera-Kitaka S, Semitala F, Mwebaze-Songa P, Castelnuovo B, Schaefer P, Spacek LA, Gasasira AF, Katabira E, Colebunders R, Quinn TC, Ronald A, Thomas DL, Kekitiinwa A: Predictors of long-term viral failure among Ugandan children and adults treated with antiretroviral therapy. J Acquir Immune Defic Syndr 2007;46:187–193.

51 Bangsberg DR: Adherence, viral suppression, and resistance to antiretroviral therapy. AIDS Reader 2007;17(suppl):S11–S15.

52 Pearson CR, Micek M, Simoni JM, Matediana E, Martin DP, Gloyd S: Modified directly observed therapy to faciliate high active antiretroviral therapy adherence in Beira, Mozambique. J Acquir Immune Defic Syndr 2006;43:S134–S141.

53 Orrell C, Harling G, Lawn SD, Kaplan R, McNally M, Bekker LG, Wood R: Conservation of first-line antiretroviral treatment regimen where therapeutic options are limited. Antivir Ther 2007;12:83–88.

54 Culbert H, Tu D, O'Brien DP, Ellman T, Mills C, Ford N, Amisi T, Chan K, Venis S: HIV treatment in a conflict setting: outcomes and experiences from Bukavu, Democratic Republic of the Congo. PLoS Med 2007;4:794–798.

55 Keiser O, Anastos K, Schechter M, Balestre E, Myer L, Boulle A, Bangsberg D, Toure H, Braitstein P, Sprinz E, Nash D, Hosseinipour M, Dabis F, May M, Brinkhof MW, Egger M: Antiretroviral therapy in resource-limited settings 1996 to 2006: patient characteristics, treatment regimens and monitoring in Sub-Saharan Africa, Asia and Latin America. Trop Med Int Health 2008;13:870–879.

56  Bisson GP, Gross R, Strom JB, Rollins C, Bellamy S, Weinstein R, Friedman H, Dickinson D, Frank I, Strom BL, Gaolathe T, Ndwapi N: Diagnostic accuracy of CD4 cell count increase for virologic response after initiating highly active antiretroviral therapy. AIDS 2006;20:1613–1619.

57  Pillay D, Kityo C, Robertson V, Lyagoba F, Dunn D, Tugume S, Hakim J, Munden P, Gilks C, Kaleebu P; DART Virology Group and Trial Team: Emergence and evolution of drug resistance in the absence of viral load monitoring during 48 weeks of combivir/tenofovir within the DART Trial. 14th Conf Retroviruses Opportunistic Infect, Los Angeles, 2007, poster 642.

58  The ART-LINC of IeDEA Study Group: Switching to second-line antiretroviral therapy in resource-limited settings: comparison of programmes with and without viral load monitoring. AIDS 2009;23:1867–1874.

59  Cozzi-Lepri A, Phillips AN, Ruiz L, Clotet B, Loveday C, Kjaer J, Mens H, Clumeck N, Viksna L, Antunes F, Machala L, Lundgren JD: Evolution of drug resistance in HIV-infected patients remaining on a virologically failing combination antiretroviral therapy regimen. AIDS 2007;21:721–732.

60  Gupta RK, Hill A, Sawyer AW, Cozzi-Lepri A, von Wyl V, Yerly S, Lima VD, Gunthard HF, Gilks C, Pillay D: Virological monitoring and resistance to first-line highly active antiretroviral therapy in adults infected with HIV-1 treated under WHO guidelines: a systematic review and meta-analysis. Lancet Infect Dis 2009;9:409–417.

61  Hosseinipour MC, van Oosterhout JJ, Weigel R, Phiri S, Kamwendo D, Parkin N, Fiscus SA, Nelson JA, Eron JJ, Kumwenda J: The public health approach to identify antiretroviral therapy failure: high-level nucleoside reverse transcriptase inhibitor resistance among Malawians failing first-line antiretroviral therapy. AIDS 2009;23:1127–1134.

62  Kouanfack C, Montavon C, Laurent C, Aghokeng A, Kenfack A, Bourgeois A, Koulla-Shiro S, Mpoudi-Ngole E, Peeters M, Delaporte E: Low levels of antiretroviral-resistant HIV infection in a routine clinic in Cameroon that uses the World Health Organization (WHO) public health approach to monitor antiretroviral treatment and adequacy with the WHO recommendation for second-line treatment. Clin Infect Dis 2009;48:1318–1322.

63  Margot NA, Enejosa J, Cheng AK, Miller MD, McColl DJ: Development of HIV-1 drug resistance through 144 weeks in antiretroviral-naive subjects on emtricitabine, tenofovir disoproxil fumarate, and efavirenz compared with lamivudine/zidovudine and efavirenz in study GS-01-934. J Acquir Immune Defic Syndr 2009;52:209–221.

64  Hosseinipour M, Kumwenda J, Weigel R, Brown L, Mzinganjira D, Mhango B, Phiri S, Van Oosterhout J: Clinical, immunological, and virological outcomes of second-line treatment, Malawi. 16th Conf Retroviruses Opportunistic Infect, Montreal, 2009. www.retroconference.org/2009/Abstracts/35596.htm (accessed January 5, 2010).

65  Renaud-Théry F, Nguimfack BD, Vitoria M, Lee E, Perriens J: Use of antiretroviral therapy in resource-limited countries in 2007: up-take of 2nd-line and paediatric treatment stagnant. XVII Int AIDS Conf, Mexico City, 2008, oral presentation THPDB103.

66  Boulle A, Orrel C, Kaplan R, Van Cutsem G, McNally M, Hilderbrand K, Myer L, Egger M, Coetzee D, Maartens G, Wood R: Substitutions due to antiretroviral toxicity or contraindication in the first 3 years of antiretroviral therapy in a large South African cohort. Antivir Ther 2007;12:753–760.

67  Johnson JA, Li J-f, Morris L, Mertinson N, Gray G, McIntyre J, Heneine W: Emergence of drug-resistant HIV-1 after intrapartum administration of single-dose nevirapine is substantially underestimated. J Infect Dis 2006;192:16–23.

68  Lockman S, Shapiro RL, Smeaton LM, Wester C, Thior Ibou, Stevens L, Chand F, Makhema J, Moffat C, Asmelash A, Ndase P, Arimi P, van Widenfelt E, Mashani L, Novitsky V, Lagakos S, and Essex M: Response to antiretroviral therapy after a single, peripartum dose of nevirapine. N Engl J Med 2007;356:135–147.

69  Arrivé E, Newell ML, Ekouevi DK, Chaix ML, Thiebaut R, Masquelier B, Leroy V, Perre PV, Rouzioux C, Dabis F: Prevalence of resistance to nevirapine in mothers and children after single-dose exposure to prevent vertical transmission of HIV-1: a meta-analysis. Int J Epidemiol 2007;36:1009–1021.

70  Mellors JW and Chow JY: Single-dose nevirapine to prevent mother-to-child transmission of HIV type 1: balancing the benefits and risks. Clin Infect Dis 2009;48:473–475.

71  Arrive E, Dabis F: Prophylactic antiretroviral regimens for prevention of mother-to-child transmission of HIV in resource-limited settings. Curr Opin HIV AIDS 2008;3:161–165.

72  Gray GE: Walking the tightrope in prevention of mother-to-child transmission of HIV infection. Clin Infect Dis 2008;46:622–624.

73  Loubser S, Balfe P, Sherman G, Hammer S, Kuhn L, Morris L: Decay of K103N mutants in cellular DNA and plasma RNA after single-dose nevirapine to reduce mother-to-child HIV transmission. AIDS 2006;20:995–1002.

74   Mandala J, Torpey K, Kasonde P, Kabaso M, Dirks R, Suzuki C, Thompson C, Sangiwa G, Mukadi YD: Prevention of mother-to-child transmission of HIV in Zambia: implementing efficacious ARV regimens in primary health centers. BMC Public Health, 2009;9:314.

75   World Health Organization: Rapid advice: use of antiretroviral drugs for treating pregnant women and preventing HIV infection in infants. 2009. www.who.int/hiv/pub/arv/rapid_advice_art.pdf (accessed December 24, 2009).

76   Dao H, Mofenson LM, Ekpini R, Gilks CF, Barnhart M, Bolu O, Shaffer N: International recommendations on antiretroviral drugs for treatment of HIV-infected women and prevention of mother-to-child HIV transmission in resource-limited settings: 2006 update. Am J Obstet Gynecol 2007;197:S42–S55.

77   World Health Organization: Report of the WHO Technical Reference Group, Paediatric HIV/ART Care Guideline Group meeting. 2008. www.who.int/hiv/pub/paediatric/WHO_Paediatric_ART_guideline_rev_mreport_2008.pdf.

78   Calmy A: Missing ARVs for HIV/AIDS treatment in 2009. UNITAID briefing at 62nd WHA, Geneva, 2009. www.msfaccess.org/fileadmin/user_upload/diseases/hiv-aids/dr.%2520calmy%2520unitaid%2520wha%2520briefing.pdf (accessed January 2, 2010).

79   Baggaley RF, Garnett GP, Ferguson NM: Modelling the Impact of antiretroviral use in resource-poor settings. PLoS Med 2006;3:e124–e136.

80   Blower S, Brodine E, Kahn J, McFarland W: The antiretroviral rollout and drug-resistant HIV in Africa: insights from empirical data and theoretical models. AIDS 2005;19:1–14.

81   Vardavas R, Blower S: The emergence of HIV transmitted resistance in Botswana: 'when will the WHO detection threshold be exceeded?'. PLoS ONE, 2007;2:e152.

82   Deeks SG: Treatment of antiretroviral-drug-resistant HIV-1 infection. Lancet 2003;362:2002–2011.

83   DART Virology Group and Trial Team: Virological response to a triple nucleoside/nucleotide analogue regimen over 48 weeks in HIV-1-infected adults in Africa. AIDS 2006;20:1391–1399.

84   Eron JJ Jr, Bartlett JA, Santana JL, Bellos NC, Johnson J, Keller A, et al: Persistent antiretroviral activity of nucleoside analogues after prolonged zidovudine and lamivudine therapy as demonstrated by rapid loss of activity after discontinuation. J Acquir Immune Defic Syndr 2004;37: 1581–1583.

85   Cornman DH, Kiene SM, Christie S, Fisher WA, Shuper PA, Pillay S, Friedland GH, Thomas CM, Lodge L, Fisher JD: Clinic-based intervention reduces unprotected sexual behavior among HIV-infected patients in KwaZulu-Natal, South Africa: results of a pilot study. J Acquir Immune Defic Syndr 2008;48:553–560.

86   Bunnell R, et al: Changes in sexual behavior and risk of HIV transmission after antiretroviral therapy and prevention interventions in rural Uganda. AIDS 2006;20:85–92.

87   Bunnell R, Mermin J, DeCock KM: HIV prevention for a threatened continent: implementing positive prevention in Africa. JAMA 2006;296:855–858.

88   World Health Organization and Joint United Nations Program on HIV/AIDS: Guidance on provider-initiated HIV Testing and counseling in health facilities. 2007. http://whqlibdoc.who.int/publications/2007/9789241595568_eng.pdf (accessed January 5, 2009).

89   Little SJ, Dawson K, Hellman NS, Richman DD, Frost SDW: Persistence of transmitted drug-resistant virus among subjects with primary HIV infection deferring antiretroviral therapy. Antiviral Ther 2004;8:S129–S129.

90   Pao D, Andrady U, Clarke J, et al: Long-term persistence of primary genotypic resistance after HIV-1 seroconversion. J Acquir Immune Defic Syndr 2004; 37:1570–1573.

91   Hue S, Gifford RJ, Dunn D, Fernhill E, Pillay D: Demonstration of sustained drug-resistant human immunodeficiency virus type 1 lineages circulating among treatment-naive individuals. J Virol 2009;83: 2645–2654.

92   Bennett DE, Bertagnolio S, Sutherland D, Gilks CF: The World Health Organization's global strategy for prevention and assessment of HIV drug resistance. Antiviral Ther 2008;13(suppl 2):1–13.

93   Jordan MR, Bennett DE, Bertagnolio S, Sutherland D, Gilks C: World Health Organization surveys to monitor HIV drug resistance prevention and associated factors in sentinel antiretroviral treatment sites. Antiviral Ther 2008;13(suppl 2):15–23.

94   Myatt M, Bennett DE: Development of a novel sequential sampling technique for the surveillance of transmitted HIV drug resistance by cross-sectional survey for use in low resource settings. Antiviral Ther 2008;13(suppl 2):19–37.

95   Bennett DE, Myatt M, Sutherland D, Bertagnolio S, Gilks CF: Recommendations for surveillance of transmitted hiv drug resistance in countries scaling up antiretroviral treatment. Antiviral Ther 2008; 13(suppl 2):25–36.

96   Ndembi N, Lyagoba R, Nanteza B, Kishemererwa G, Serwanga J, Katongole-Mbidde E, Grosskuth H, Kaleebu P: Transmitted antiretroviral drug resistance surveillance among newly HIV type 1-diagnosed women attending an antenatal clinic in Entebbe, Uganda. AIDS Res Hum Retroviruses 2008;24:889–895.

97   Laurent C, Kouanfack C, Koulla-Shiro S, et al: Effectiveness and safety of a generic fixed-dose combination of nevirapine, stavudine, and lamivudine in HIV-1 infected adults in Cameroon: open-label multicentre trial. Lancet, 2004;364:29–34.

98 UNITAID: UNITAID approves patent pool. 2009. www.unitaid.eu/en/20091215237/News/UNITAID-APPROVES-PATENT-POOL.html (accessed January 19, 2010).

99 Nachega J, Stein DM, Lehman DA, et al: Adherence to antiretroviral therapy in HIV-infected adults in Soweto, South Africa. AIDS Hum Retroviruses 2004;20:1053–1057.

100 Dlamini PS, Wantland D, Makoae LN, Chirwa M, Kohi TW, Greeff M, Naidoo J, Mullan J, Uys LR, Holzemer WL: HIV stigma and missed medications in HIV-positive people in five African countries. AIDS Patient Care STDS 2009;23:377–387.

101 Liamputtong P, Haritavorn N, Kiatying-Angsulee N: HIV and AIDS, stigma and AIDS support groups: perspectives from women living with HIV and AIDS in central Thailand. Soc Sci Med 2009;69:862–868.

102 Jha CK, Madison J: Disparity in health care: HIV, stigma, and marginalization in Nepal. J Int AIDS Soc 2009;12:16.

103 Gamper A, Nathaniel S, Robbe IJ: Universal access to antiretroviral therapy and HIV stigma in Botswana. Am J Public Health 2009;99:968–969.

104 Zhou J, Phanupak P, Kiertiburanakul S, Ditangco R, Kamarulzaman A, Pujary S: Highly active antiretroviral treatment containing efavirenz or nevirapine and related toxicity in the TREAT Asia HIV Observational Database. J Acquir Immune Defic Syndr 2006;43:501–503.

105 Nuesch R, Srasuebkul P, Ananworanich J, Ruxrungtham K, Phanuphak P, Duncombe C: Monitoring the toxicity of antiretroviral therapy in resource limited settings: a prospective clinical trial cohort in Thailand. J Antimicrob Chemother 2006;58:637–644.

Diane E. Bennett
Global AIDS Program
Centers for Disease Control and Prevention
Atlanta GA 30329 (USA)
Tel. +1 404 649 5349/+41 22 791 5066, E-Mail dbennett@cdc.gov and bennettd@who.int

# Author Index

# Subject Index